STOP YOUR
NECK PAIN AND HEADACHE NOW

STOP YOUR
NECK PAIN AND HEADACHE NOW

Fast and Safe Relief in Minutes
Proven Effective for Thousands of Patients

Rowlin L. Lichter, M.D.
Board-Certified Orthopedic Surgeon

iUniverse, Inc.
Bloomington

Stop Your Neck Pain and Headache Now
Fast and Safe Relief in Minutes
Proven Effective for Thousands of Patients

iUniverse books may be ordered through booksellers or by contacting:

iUniverse
1663 Liberty Drive
Bloomington, IN 47403
www.iuniverse.com
1-800-Authors (1-800-288-4677)

ISBN: 978-1-4620-4578-5 (sc)
ISBN: 978-1-4620-4579-2 (hc)
ISBN: 978-1-4620-4580-8 (ebk)

Printed in the United States of America

iUniverse rev. date: 10/20/2011

CONTENTS

What Is Your Problem?

What Can You Do?

What Else Can You Do?

Marketing Headline

STOP YOUR NECK PAIN AND HEADACHE NOW with simple, painless, non-surgical techniques. Fast and safe relief in just minutes a day. Proven effective by thousands for over thirty years. Medically-approved methods are yours without a prescription.

Key Words

Neck; Self-help; Pain; Headache; Neckache; Spasm; Treatment; Non-surgical; Holistic; Cervical Spine; Whiplash; Tension; Exercise; Causes of neck pain and headache; Stop the Pain Immediately; Self-help treatments; Physical therapy; Neck and head pain prevention; Questionable treatments; Choosing a doctor; Fast pain relief; Active treatment; Passive treatment; Orthopedic; Osteopathic; Physical medicine; Physiatrist; Neck anatomy; Neck physiology; Ergonomics; Arthritis; TMD; HNP; Slipped disc; Massage; Stretches; Chiropractic; Acupuncture; Stress; Complementary and Alternative Medicine.

Biography

Rowlin L. Lichter, M.D., FAAOS, FNASS, FABS, is a board-certified orthopedic surgeon trained at Northwestern University with over sixty years of clinical experience. After practicing in Hawaii and Nevada, he now donates orthopedic services to the underserved in Reno.

Dr. Lichter established the prestigious CHART Rehabilitation Centers of Hawaii in 1979 and pioneered the use of sports medicine methods with physical therapy and work conditioning.

His five children are scattered from Hawaii to Colorado. His wife of almost fifty years, Barbara, supports and guides him and shares his hobbies of food, wine, travel and writing.

Forward

Ten minutes a day can end your neck pain, and I'll throw in headache relief, too.

Stop Your Neck Pain and Headache Now offers an effective remedy which I have personally tested and found successful in my clinical practice.

Stress is the major cause of neck pain and headaches. Almost everyone has stress and has had a pain in the neck at one time or another. Most often you can get your pain-in-the-neck to bug off. When you cannot get rid of your stress or the pain is from another correctable cause, I am here to help, so continue reading.

I have been a bone doctor, an orthopedic surgeon and clinician, for perhaps too many years, teaching sufferers how to stop their neck pain and headaches quickly and easily. Popping a pill is not the answer. It usually offers only temporary relief, and then you need another pill and soon you need more or stronger medicine. *All* medicines can be poisons, so why tempt fate? Complementary and alternative medicine (CAM therapies), like acupuncture and the many kinds of massage and shiatsu, may be effective but they give only temporary relief.

I have worked side by side with pioneers of effective surgical treatment of neck problems. Surgery has proven to be a valid option, but it is the final option. This book is dedicated to avoiding that option if at all possible.

Conservative treatment concepts became attractive in my early years of practice. These techniques have been used and practiced for more than thirty years in the active physical rehabilitation centers that I developed. The treatments became more practical and easier to use with the help of my therapists at CHART Rehabilitation in Hawaii. CHART is an acronym for Comprehensive Health and Rehabilitation Training. The clinics are outpatient physical and occupational therapy centers for musculoskeletal problems. CHART therapists teach people how to get and stay well. Internal research and tracking proved these methods to be eighty-five per cent successful in treating headache and neck problems. These methods have been copied in most of the advanced and current physical therapy offices in the United States and elsewhere. Now, doctors and therapists all over the world have followed my lead and adopted these methods, confirming the techniques' effectiveness. This cure is yours without a prescription!

And, do not stop following my instructions just because you feel great. Integrate what you learn from this book into your normal healthy lifestyle.

Even if you are one of the fifteen per cent I cannot help, I will tell you what you need to do next.

The chapters address different aspects of head and neck problems, including their correction. However, this is not an exhaustive documentation or a scientific treatise on the subject of head and neck pain. It is simply the result of treating patients with head and neck pain for the past sixty-three years.

A good and cooperative patient must understand the problem he or she needs to overcome and how the treatment should work. I have attempted to explain as clearly as possible with only a few medical terms just how the neck and its connected parts are put together and how they work.

Many things can go wrong with the human body and its delicately balanced mechanisms. However, this book is limited to problems of the neck, head, upper back and shoulders.

You can do many things to help your body restore normal function. An entire chapter is devoted to those general actions that will reduce head and neck pain.

Currently, exercise is the closest thing to a panacea of healing. Extremely effective exercises describe and illustrate how to control neck and head pain of musculoskeletal origin within minutes. Further methods guide the reader to prolong or permanently extend that relief.

No remedy works for everyone. I offer the reader alternatives to what I have found to be the most effective therapies. The more common choices of healers are described and critiqued, giving the reader an idea of what treatments are available.

I admit to my training bias. Medical doctors are men of Science. We are trained to look with disfavor on and to be aware of unproven techniques and philosophies. These methods are discussed as objectively as possible in a separate chapter. If you choose one of these unscientific methods, you will be able to do it with a clearer vision of what to expect.

The penultimate chapter tells what to expect when seeing a competent practitioner of each of the most commonly-accepted healing regimens.

Acknowledgments

I am profoundly grateful to the professional staff of CHART Rehabilitation of Hawaii for its helpful reviews and additions.

Special thanks go to the late Dr. Vert Mooney, teacher, scientist and author, for his pioneering work in active physical rehabilitation and his encouragement of my work. He nurtured my interest and growth in this field.

I am deeply indebted to my wife, Barbara, for her meaningful and patient help. A sweeter, more intelligent, loving and beautiful pain in the neck has never blessed any man for forty-eight wonderful years, and counting.

Disclaimer

These self-help tips can relieve and prevent *most* common neck, head and upper back problems with maximum safety. These methods have been used successfully in Comprehensive Health and Rehabilitation Training (CHART) physical therapy centers for thousands of patients without complications.

Please review and understand the cautions regarding exercise in Chapter 7. Rare situations and unusual individuals do exist. For example, the sudden onset of a severe headache, with or without neck stiffness, can be a symptom of a serious, even fatal, condition. A physician must evaluate the problem immediately.

If you are not sure about the safety and appropriateness of the suggestions in this book, ask your doctor. If any of the suggestions are not helping, please seek medical help. You may have a more serious problem.

If you are under a physician's care, discuss the advisability of following the self-care advice in this book.

Chapter 1

The Inside Story: Anatomy 101

(Possibly More Than You Wanted to Know)

*The head bone connects to the neck bone, and the neck bone
connects to another neck bone . . .
Not quite the way the song goes.*

It helps to know the subject. You get well faster when you understand the problem. However, in medical school anatomy was never much fun, so I will make these descriptions as simple and painless as possible. If you are not in the didactic mood, skip to Chapter 4, Basic Concepts.

Neck Bones and Spinal Cord

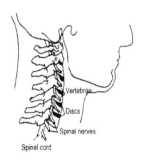

Bones, Spinal Nerves and Discs

The head is like a twelve-pound bowling ball sitting on top of seven construction blocks strung together by the ligaments and muscles. The neck moves the head, balances it over the shoulders and lets us turn our heads in any direction but backward (except for the Stephen King models). The neck moves the head to keep our eyes pointed where we want to see and our ears turned the right direction. The neck bones surround the spinal cord which extends from the brain to the rest of the body. The spinal cord has the consistency of cooked pasta, firm (al dente), so it must have bony protection. Nerves exit between the neck bones on each side of the spine and spread out like branches on a tree in the neck to the rest of your upper body.

The neck muscles are placed so that they usually avoid hitting, bending or stretching these nerves, but poor or long-held unusual postures can cause pressure on the structures resulting in pain.

Discs and Spinal Nerves

The rubbery spacers between the neck bones are called discs. They have an outer casing (annulus) of fibrous tissue that is laced with natural fibers crisscrossed like a radial automobile tire. There is a tough, jelly-like center called the nucleus pulposus. It is normally only a little harder than the dried-out film on old gelatin.

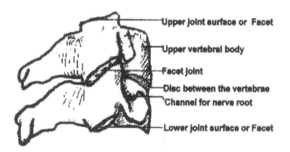

A Motion Segment

A disc attaches to each saucer-shaped top and slightly rounded bottom surface of a neck bone. The discs cushion every step we take. Without these cushions, the force of stepping off a curb would be transmitted up the spinal column and could literally knock you unconscious.

Discs hold the neck bones apart, allowing free passage of the spinal nerves that emerge between each spinal segment. When the neck bends forward, the back sides of the bones separate farther and make more room for the nerves to pass.

2

The disc has a pair of weak spots where the nerves pass. A blow out or rupture here can damage or irritate the nerve. This is termed a ruptured intervertebral disc, commonly called a slipped disc. Since the interior of the disc, the nucleus pulposus, herniates, the herniated nucleus pulposus becomes an HNP in medical shorthand.

Joints

The neck joints, like almost all other joints, are lined with slick resilient cartilage and filled with a fluid that allows smooth, low-friction movement. The cartilage also cushions the bone against sudden impacts. You can get some idea of how tough the neck is just watching boxing, football, hockey or other contact sports. Of course, these are dedicated athletes who have developed super strong protective neck muscles, have maintained excellent flexibility and wear protective devices like the horse collar. Still, with all these preparations, serious neck injuries do occur even to these professional players.

Ligaments

Neck ligaments control the range of movements through the disc and the spinal (facet) joints and they limit overall ranges of neck movement. They are strong, string-like structures that span the joints. The ligaments, the joint and muscle coverings (fascia) and the muscles hold the neck bones in place. A large spinal ligament limits forward bending of the neck as a whole. Medicalese is not always esoteric. This is an easy one to understand. This ligament is called the ligament of the neck; but in Latin, of course, it is called the Ligamentum Nuchae.

Fascia

Sheets of very tough material called fascia surround each muscle and bind larger muscle groups together. Wide sheets of thick fascia limit motion and connect muscles over large regions, such as the neck to the shoulders or the entire back to the pelvis.

Muscles

The neck bends and twists smoothly. Although joint capsules and ligaments limit the neck's motion and help keep the head from just flopping around, there are thirty-two muscles that control movement of the head, neck and shoulders.

Neck muscles constantly work with nerve reflexes that instantly tighten and loosen the muscles to keep the head and eyes aimed in the right direction. Take a few steps and see how complicated it is to keep your head steady while simply walking.

Neck and Upper Back Muscles

The trapezius is the largest muscle in the neck-upper back region. The muscle is a huge diamond-shape that extends from shoulder to shoulder and from the base of the skull to the waist line. The trapezius, along with several layers of muscles beneath it, moves the shoulder blades, head and spine.

The muscles in the front of the neck and upper chest are smaller and weaker than those in the back. These muscles bend your head and neck forward. They tilt your head from side to side and turn it right and left. The muscles in the front of the neck rarely contribute to chronic or long-lasting neck pain.

Superhighway of the Neck and Its Branches

All of your blood travels to and from your brain in blood vessels on the sides of your windpipe and in another set of blood vessels that passes inside the neck bones through a narrow opening in the top of the chest.

All the air to your lungs passes through the windpipe in your neck. All we eat and drink passes down our necks through the esophagus.

Other important things go through and/or stay in your neck. This includes lymph vessels and lymph glands, thyroid and parathyroid glands, some nerves and voice box (larynx).

Chapter 2

How Your Neck Should Work

Whoever called it necking was a poor judge of anatomy . . .
Groucho Marx (1895-1977)

The Biologic (not Bionic) Machine

Many people, even your doctor, compare the human body with a machine. They are only partly right. Man-made things of metal and plastic wear out as they are used. The more you drive, the sooner your tires wear out. Men build machines with extra strength and precision to delay their inevitable breakdown from wear and tear. When a machine breaks, someone has to fix it. When a machine starts to fail, the last thing you want to do is make it work harder.

The human body, however, is a biologic machine. Biologic machines can and will fix themselves if given half a chance. Most often, the repair is more than adequate. With only a little help, such as a little extra rest or proper use, the repair is successful.

Pain and Improved Function

After injury a biologic machine must be used for proper healing, although activity may hurt. For example, a scar forms as a muscle heals. The scar shrinks or contracts and the shortening could be permanently limiting. To prevent this, we must use the muscle while it is healing and keep the scar stretched. Using torn ligaments and broken bones during the healing phase actually helps restore their normal function.

Ligament fibers line up in a more normal position when they are used during healing. Even the internal structure of the bone re-forms best when bone regrowth is guided by use during the healing process.

The exercise cliché, "No pain, no gain," is only partly true and following that advice blindly can be dangerous. Mild discomfort is probably essential for proper healing of an injured neck, but over doing things is more painful and can result in further injury. Carefully and cautiously directing stresses to the muscles, bones and ligaments helps them heal stronger. Stressing an area to make it stronger or simply to maintain its integrity may be uncomfortable, but this is how we *talk* to our bodies. The body must be challenged to improve its function or to restore normal function of an injured part. The challenge is progressive use beyond current abilities. Stressing neck and shoulder muscles just enough to make them stronger is beneficial and is called the "training effect." The art is to increase function without overuse and can be guided only by listening to your body.

Pain lasting long after exercise is a warning sign. A muscular and boney structure like your neck may hurt during or shortly after almost any stressful use. If the activity causes pain to linger, reduce the intensity and duration of your activity. Consult your physician if discomfort does not go away.

"Pushing through an injury" translates into "I do not care how much it hurts; I am going to do it anyway." This approach is almost always wrong. Such an attitude demands professional oversight (or sometimes a psychiatrist).

A reasonable rule of thumb is: If it still hurts the following morning after you have been up and around an hour or so and after a warm shower or bath, you have done too much. You should rest actively, of course, until your comfort returns.

This rule is not perfect, but it works for most of us. If pain persists, you may need professional help or guidance.

Muscles and Voluntary Control

Emotions, such as fear or anxiety, begin in the brain and are the most difficult to control causes of excessive muscle tension. The mind can upset the balanced controls of muscle movement. Emotions can amplify, veto or even completely change the intended regulation of muscle tension.

There are two peripheral nervous systems. The voluntary system is the one we control and consciously perceive and react to. It allows us to move muscles and feel heat, cold, pressure, etc. The other nervous system called the sympathetic, involuntary or vegetative nervous system runs the peripheral machinery of life. It controls, among other things, the blood vessel sizes and blood flow, the lung air passages, sweating, reaction of the eyes to light, subtle growth and repair processes and the fear response called fight or flight. It even controls or mediates pain. A clash of the voluntary and the sympathetic nervous systems results in a chronic fight or flight response and a stiff neck amongst other changes. Nonetheless, properly directed, this central control of muscle tension can be an important therapeutic tool. For example, the ISOMAGIC exercises described later in this book and conscious relaxation will help quiet some of the detrimental, excessive responses of the sympathetic nerves.

Muscle Injuries

When one muscle contracts, the opposing muscle(s) must relax to allow movement. This is called reciprocal innervation and normally allows for smoother rather than jerky motions. Defects in this reciprocal innervation, the suppression of one movement as the opposite one occurs, can cause pain and injury as one muscle improperly opposes the other. Sudden repeated actions can interfere with this essential reaction and cause the muscle to tear itself apart. Relaxation is a key to avoid this. Exercise can correct this. Do not omit the warm up before exercise.

A muscle rarely contracts completely but it reacts in small bundles. Some bundles tighten while others relax and restore their glycogen fuel. This lets the muscle remain tense for a longer time. A weak muscle can perform strongly for a short time if it uses more muscle units at a time than normally. This overuse could seriously injure that muscle by tearing itself apart.

Neck muscles can be overused by heavy lifting, a sudden fright or a rear-end car accident. This is called a muscle strain. Even after resting the injured muscle, it may be too seriously injured to continue working normally and may need time to heal. Use it sparingly while it heals.

Use Your Bones

Bone is a living tissue. Bone can become stronger or weaker according to how hard and how much we use it. If you do not use your bones, they become thin and are easier to break. Use your neck bones with regular exercise, and they will get stronger and more resistant to injury.

Remember that bone needs calcium for strength and stiffness or resistance to breaking. Calcium is also essential for muscle contraction and other cell functions. If dietary calcium is inadequate, your body robs it from the bones. Be sure that you have enough calcium in your diet with dairy foods and leafy vegetables or calcium supplements. And, do not forget to get enough vitamin D to control the use of calcium.

Normal Posture

Good posture prevents and corrects many neck problems. Your head must be balanced properly to prevent straining the neck muscles. The shape of the spinal bones and the arrangement of their supporting structures (ligaments, joints, fascia and muscles) favor bending straight forward and backward. To bend sideward or to rotate, the complicated mechanical linkage in the spine makes front-to-back curves necessary in the neck and also in the lower back.

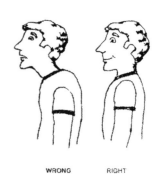

WRONG   RIGHT

Your neck has a forward curve which partly balances the backward curve of the chest region. The two forward curves of the neck and lower back should exactly balance the backward curve of the chest region.

Abnormal Posture

Standing or sitting with bad posture can cause a chronic muscle strain and create a serious pain problem. Leaning too far forward puts a strain on the back of the neck and bending too far backward pulls on the muscles in front of the neck.

The curve in the neck flattens or reverses with injury, since all the neck muscles tighten to hold the painful area still. This results in an imbalance which leads to a strain, and the strain causes pain. This makes maintaining good posture more difficult, yet more important.

The imbalance is not restricted to the neck. If one part of your spine is too straight or too curved, the others must compensate. If one curve is extreme, both it and the compensating curves may be sources of pain.

Good Posture and Swayback

Good posture begins at the bottom. If your bottom sticks out too much behind you, it is a sure sign of too much sway in your back. Swayback can result from poor standing posture which often is seen in people with flat feet. If your back is badly swayed, this may be a significant and correctable cause of your neck pain.

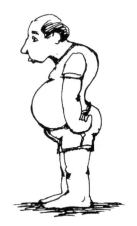

Try this swayback test. Stand with your back close against a wall with both your buttocks and shoulders touching lightly. Do not move and gently press your hand behind the small of your back. If the curve of your back is normal, you can probably slip only four fingers of your hand between your back and the wall without moving away. If

Swayback

9

your hand slides between your back and the wall easily, you are either swaybacked or are overweight or both. Neither is good for your neck.

Next, find a hard, straight-backed chair to check your seated posture. Use the chair as you would the wall. Sit up straight. Slide your buttocks against the chair back. Lean backward until your shoulders also touch. Then, without moving away from the chair back, again try to slide your hand behind your back. The conclusions are the same.

Some curves are fixed and cannot be changed. To maintain balance, there must be curves above and below that balance the abnormal one(s). These adjacent curves are flexible and can be corrected to some degree. Scoliosis is a fixed developmental, sideward curve of the spine. It may involve the neck, but occurs here less often than in the rest of the spine. This is almost exclusively a female problem. Most of the curves are minor and are not a significant cause of neck pain. However, rarely, these curves can complicate neck problems. When they do, you will need medical advice to combat their complications.

Occasionally, a sideward spinal curve may develop suddenly, within hours or days. This may be a musculoskeletal problem from injury or overuse. However, if you do not recall a significant injury, something more serious may be making your muscles pull you out of balance. In an adult's neck, it is most often due to an infection in the ear, mouth or throat and only rarely in the neck. This needs immediate medical attention.

Chapter 3

What Causes Neck Pain?

What Can Go Wrong?

Two wrongs don't make a right . . . English proverb

Overuse or Improper Use

Overuse or abuse is the most common cause of minor neck pain. Weekend athletes are good examples. Five days of sitting around cannot prepare you for a weekend of overuse without risking injury. You should include at least one other day of exercise mid-week. Do not try to prove that you are in better shape than you really are while playing on the weekend. Muscles that are not accustomed to heavy use may break, tear or severely cramp. Joints that are stiff from sitting all week are more easily sprained.

The springtime house cleaner is another potential abuser. Doing all the hard and heavy work over just a few days leads to injury. Plan your assault on the annual chores. Spread the stress over days or even weeks, as suited to your or your help's abilities.

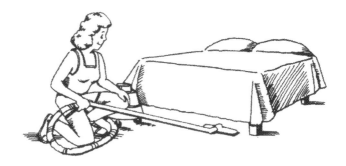

When you exercise, your muscles need fuel. The basic fuel is glycogen which is a breakdown product derived from complex dietary sugars and starches. When glycogen is burned too rapidly by your muscles for the available oxygen, lactic acid is produced. With overuse this irritating chemical builds up faster than the body can get rid of it, causing muscle pain. Final breakdown to carbon dioxide and water removes the lactic acid completely, but this takes some time. If stiffness or soreness after exercise lasts longer than a day, you have done too much. Rest a day and next time cut back. However, if the chemical irritation is mild, transient discomfort can be beneficial. This is the "training effect," which leads to muscle strengthening. Ice, heat, massage, stretching and some electrical treatments used by professionals, such as electrical stimulation and interferential stimulation of the muscle to create relaxation, can rapidly relax the muscles and make you feel good sooner.

Muscle Spasm or Tension

True muscle spasms are much rarer than professionals identify them. Usually the muscles are simply tight. Tight muscles result from a failure to voluntarily relax them. This is the tension that causes most tension head and neck aches. Under tension or apprehension primitive muscular reflexes mimic the effect of a threatened physical attack, tightening the muscles one would use to fight off an attacker. Fear of an individual, fear of failure and insecurity, as in addressing a crowd or not meeting a deadline, or the many challenges of daily living frequently activate these neck reflexes. After prolonged tension lactic acid irritation causes even more muscle tension. Prolonged punishment like this can cause shortening of muscles that may require weeks to restore to normal length.

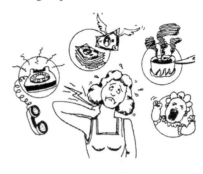

Meanwhile, chronic tension subtly changes the brain and nervous system, heightening reflexes and sharpening sensation. Besides overuse, some other causes of tight muscles are poor circulation, direct muscle injury, disease and a sprain or fracture.

The Worry Wort

Minor Muscle Tears

A muscle tear is a strain. This should not be confused with a stretched or partially torn ligament which is a sprain. A muscle can contract so strongly that it tears itself apart. Sudden stresses without a proper warm-up are a common cause of a muscle tear. Even sudden turning or stretching of the head and neck could result in a minor tear. The best prevention is warming up before exercise. However, if you cannot avoid injury, use the first aid techniques in Chapter 5.

Whiplash or Acceleration/Deceleration Injuries

The neck is quite mobile and has an approximately twelve-pound head on top of it. As a result, the neck is frequently injured by external forces. A sudden backward force like an uppercut to the jaw or an auto accident cannot be countered quickly or adequately by the weak muscles in the front of the average neck. Minor tearing may occur in the muscles of the front of the neck in a severe rear-end auto accident. When a muscle is torn, it bleeds. Blood irritates the muscle. Blood in a muscle has to be removed by local circulation and may require about a week.

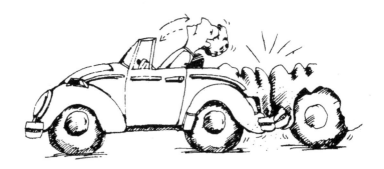

Researchers have recorded that a dead stop in a car traveling just five miles per hour can bring out complaints of significant neck pain. A rear-end auto collision causes a sudden forward blow from the car seat to the passenger's back. This impact propels most of the body forward, momentarily leaving the head behind. Before the neck muscles can react and pull the head forward, the head has dropped too far backward, straining muscles and spraining joints. The disc can break, and some inside "jelly" from the nucleus may spill out like the blowout of an automobile tire. Extreme force may tear ligaments, crush discs, break bones and injure or dislocate joints. A properly positioned head rest may minimize the stress on the neck. Ruling out all the possible neck injuries following rear-end accidents rapidly escalates the cost of emergency care.

Diving accidents, blows to the head, falls, trampoline accidents and many other sources of external force can cause similar problems. Individuals who often are subjected to these forces, such as wrestlers and football linemen, must increase the strength of their neck muscles. Usually these athletes' necks are disguised by extreme muscular development.

Jaw Joint Problems or Temporomandibular Dysfunction

A frequent cause of neck and head pain may come from the jaw joint. Dentists are aware that as many as three-quarters of all adults have actual or potential problems in the jaw or temporomandibular joint. This problem is called "Temporomandibular Dysfunction" or TMD. Poorly aligned teeth often cause chewing problems and TMD. Poor alignment may come from improper

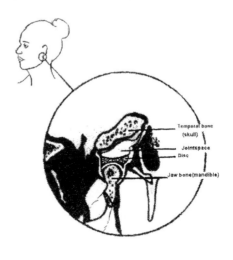

Temporomandibular Joint

growth, dental braces, fractures, bad fillings or poor nutrition. Teeth may have been lost, especially the back ones; and the remaining ones can migrate, resulting in misfit teeth or a poor bite, the way the teeth fit together. Bad habits, such as grinding the teeth (bruxism) or clenching, or direct injuries to the jaw and its joints also may cause problems. These changes cause clicking, local pain, difficulty opening the mouth widely, locking of the jaw joints and, especially, neck pain and headache. TMD also may cause ringing in the ears, occasional dizziness, and even vague arm pain is frequently associated with neck injury. Injury may occur by the jaw flying open uncontrollably during the impact or by reactively biting too hard during an accident.

Perhaps the most important source of TMD pain is emotional tension which affects the jaw joint. This tension causes the appropriately called tension headaches. The clenching and grinding of the teeth that aggravate a dysfunctional joint are directly related to emotional tension. Former cigarette smokers who substitute chewing gum for that habit also may aggravate TMD. In these cases relaxation is a prime therapeutic tool. Remember to tell your dentist about persistent headaches. He may be able to help.

15

Slipped Disc

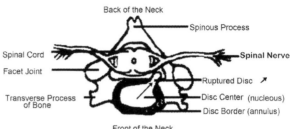

An intervertebral disc can cause trouble by its closeness to a spinal nerve. In 1933 Dr. Harvey Cushing, a famous neurosurgeon, coined the term *ruptured* disc. He noted that this abnormal disc caused severe back pain and that the pain could be relieved by surgical removal of the offending portion of the disc. Since that time discs have captured the interest and sometimes the imagination of many spinal surgeons. Remember, there are five discs to rupture in the neck; but this most often occurs between the fourth and sixth vertebrae.

The center of every healthy disc contains material that can irritate the spinal nerves if it gets into the spinal canal. When the ring (annulus) surrounding the disc breaks, the central material (nucleus pulposus) ruptures into the spinal canal, irritating the nearest nerves. This is technically a herniated nucleus pulposus or HNP. The chemical irritation from the herniation may last for many weeks.

The disc also can cause mechanical trouble when part of it pushes into the opening where the nerve passes through the vertebra. The pressure pinches the nerve and interrupts its transmission, resulting in weakness and/or numbness and/or hypersensitivity. Something normally uncomfortable, like extremes of motion, may become painful in one direction or another.

Most disc symptoms are self-limited. The body absorbs the offending material, or the nerve stops working and producing sensations of pain. But, this may take as long as two years. Therefore, sharp, burning pain, numbness or weakness is a good reason to see your doctor. He may be able to help shorten the recovery time.

Arthritis

The term arthritis simply means that the joint has been inflamed or irritated. Following are the most common types:

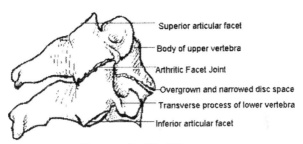

Superior articular facet

Body of upper vertebra

Arthritic Facet Joint

Overgrown and narrowed disc space

Transverse process of lower vertebra

Inferior articular facet

Degenerative Disc Disease

Degenerative Arthritis

Degenerative disc disease and/or degenerative arthritis or osteoarthritis rarely cause serious neck problems by themselves. The disc begins to change or degenerate in your teens, so effects are present and visible in most people by their mid-thirties. A little less motion and occasional aches can be expected, but the effects usually are minimal. Most doctors and other scientists associate this condition with aging. Some, however, feel it may be preventable in the future.

Getting old is only for the brave; but, as the adage goes, it is better than the alternative. Getting old gracefully is even more difficult. You can be devastated by the painful joints of osteoarthritis, also called wear-and-tear arthritis. Osteoarthritis is rarely totally crippling, but it can be a true pain in the neck. The discs in your neck wear and become thinner and less elastic. The thinning disc adds to your neck stiffness. The joints lose their smooth cartilaginous surfaces and resentfully creak and crackle. Joints begin to widen with boney outgrowths.

When degenerated discs and neck pain occur together, it is usually in older people who are less active and who act their age. Acting your age is a trap. It is a social concept that is not dictated by the passing of years. Pay no attention to it. Reducing your activities because exercise hurts is an easy dead end, resulting in lowering one's strength and ranges of motion. Settling down to act your age is not good for your health. Act as young as you feel and your body will allow. Stay that way as long as you can. Remember, if you act old, you will feel old, no matter what the calendar says. For most people, the reverse is equally true. Stay young, stay strong and stay flexible. Exercise! Think young! Activity counteracts and delays many of the effects of aging. Keep active and the degenerative changes will affect you less.

As yet, there is no cure for osteoarthritis. But you have a choice. Great advice continues to be "Move it or lose it." Necksercises will definitely help.

Traumatic Arthritis

Injury can worsen the symptoms of osteoarthritis. The increased pain may last for weeks, or it can become permanent. Injury, such as a severe whiplash sprain or a fracture in a diving accident, also can cause arthritis. This is called traumatic arthritis. An extreme mechanical force can sprain or even break a neck joint, but more often it will only injure the joint surfaces. The exact injury is difficult to diagnose and is difficult to cure. Traumatic arthritis responds well to exercise and acts like osteoarthritis, from mild to cripplingly severe.

Systemic Arthritis

There are many more forms of joint disease. Rheumatoid arthritis, for example, is an auto-immune, systemic disease that affects all the joints and even internal organs. Gout is a metabolic disease that happens when the body cannot handle uric acid, and joints become inflamed by the deposits of uric acid crystals. These diseases need a different approach than this book affords and are not appropriate for discussion here. Some, thankfully, are rare enough not to belong in this book. We will not even mention their esoteric names that often cover the fact that we do not know much about them. However, exercises would continue to be an important part of their treatment.

Outlet Syndrome

There is still another way poor posture can cause neck pain and numbness. Weakness in the muscles that support the shoulders can be a serious and painful problem. Shoulders do not have a strong boney support. The arm and shoulder blade actually hang on the chest and are held out to the side by the tiny, weak and poorly-connected collar bone or clavicle. Otherwise, only muscles support the entire upper limb. If the muscles are weak, the shoulder drops and drags on the nerves and blood vessels as they leave the neck through the thoracic outlet, causing neck and arm pain.

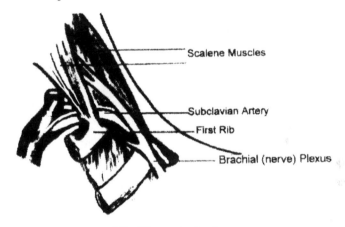

Scalene Muscles

Subclavian Artery

First Rib

Brachial (nerve) Plexus

The Thoracic Outlet

The cure is obvious. Make your muscles stronger. Restore your strength and proper posture by concentrating on neck and shoulder resistance exercises. If you have the luxuries of time and money, following instructions in a circuit weight training program for the upper body at your local gym could be beneficial. If you need more help, a personal trainer or a physical therapist can help you control this problem in about six weeks. You can expect a permanent cure in about twice that time.

Rowlin L. Lichter, M.D.

Osteoporosis

Bones gradually weaken and break without adequate calcium. This is called osteoporosis. It is caused by poor calcium nutrition, lack of exercise and deficient female hormones in women. No. That is not redundant, since men also normally manufacture female hormones. Osteoporosis rarely may cause a neck problem by itself, but the condition can explain apparent over-reaction to a supposedly minor neck injury. X-rays most often tell the tale by showing a lighter density of the bone. Your doctor can help control the problem. Osteoporosis in men is rare.

Referred Neck Pain and Headache

The source of pain is not always where you feel it. We are learning painfully slowly about pain referral and pain reflexes. The pun is intended. Our biologic machine has some built-in problems. The chemicals and electric impulses that carry pain messages in one area can leak into nearby nerve pathways. These neighboring nerves may carry the sensation to areas far away from the original pain source. However, since these adjacent nerves are being chemically stimulated, they give the false impression that the pain is coming from the region that the secondary nerve supplies. Since the pain is referred to somewhere other than where the problem started, it is called a referred pain. Most often, the remote pain will gradually decrease as the primary cause subsides.

For example, irritation of the disc or joints between the fourth and fifth neck bones causes pain between the upper edge of the shoulder blade and the spine. Pain at these areas is very common, since the joints between vertebra four and vertebra five usually are the first joints to develop neck arthritis. Irritating the discs above the fourth cervical vertebra causes pain in the back of the neck and a headache at the base of the skull. The locations of referred pain in the shoulder and upper extremity are so specific that knowing where the pain is felt, doctors often can tell the exact location of its source. If we know that, we know where to begin our treatment.

Chronic Pain Syndrome

If pain continues long after the source is gone, it is called a chronic pain syndrome. Standard chemical messengers of pain may build up around the nerves leading to and from the pain source without completely dissipating. The buildup of these messengers can make the pain persist. This way pain itself can be the cause of more pain.

Chronic pain syndrome is very hard to treat. Avoid this problem by fighting the cause of the pain before it becomes chronic. Therefore, avoid treatment that merely palliates and habituates you to repetitive treatments but does not progressively relieve your problem.

Once pain becomes chronic due to neglect, poor treatment, bad advice or other confounding factors, it is necessary to reduce one's attention to pain and refocus on function. The exercises and advice in this book will help restore function. Remember, if it functions despite pain, the problem is usually only the pain itself. *You* must refocus your attention from pain to function. Psychological help may be useful.

Chapter 4

Basic Concepts

A journey of a thousand miles begins with the first step . . .
Lao-Tzu

Your body has built-in systems to keep it normal. With a little help you can harness these actions to relieve your pain and make your neck work like it should.

1. **Rest Actively**
    Resting may be good advice in the wrong place. Do not stop everything and vegetate. Move it, even if it hurts. Plant yourself and you lose function. The need for activity despite other physical problems is close to an absolute medical necessity.

2. **Stay Active**
    Change how you act. Do not stop your activities. Use your aching muscles and joints to do ISOMAGIC and other Necksercises. Work smart and avoid dangerous stresses, but do not stop.

3. **Be Holistic**
    Holistic refers to the physical, mental and spiritual health of the whole person. Some doctors forget holistic care in order to be more efficient, focusing on just the disease. You are not just a neck. It is part of all of your body. Check all the facets of your life.

4.   **Use It or Lose It**

Enjoy the comfort of massage and manipulation if you have time and money, but you won't heal any faster. The secret is that *you* must do it. Move. You won't regret that initial twinge of discomfort, because the next move will feel better, and so on.

5.   **Stand and Sit Proud**

Sit, stand, and even lie down like the world is watching. If you look like a slob, you will feel like one. Poor posture strains your neck (and elsewhere), making it hurt.

6.   **Relax**

Work to control the tensions in your life. I know, life *is* unavoidably tense, especially your life. Tension causes tight and tired muscles which cause more muscle tension and pain. Before you employ a psychiatrist, try my simple solutions for relieving tension. You may save time and money.

7.   **Do Not Harm Yourself**

Start new or demanding physical activities involving your sore neck in small doses. Increase activities gradually. Forget "No strain, no gain." That old adage is just an invitation to injury. Talk with your body and listen to it. It is the only one you have.

8.   **Cool It**

Remember, ice is your friend for relieving acute pain. Do it right, and ice will relieve pain while relaxing tight muscles.

9.   **Pills Are Not the Answer**

All drugs can be poisons. You knew that. Use pills with care and moderation. They reduce pain but can damage your stomach, liver and kidneys. Stay organic if you wish, and avoid chemicals but only where it makes good sense. "Chemicals" and "organic" are both poorly-described terms. Do not avoid medications that may allow you to return to healthy activity and, thus, avoid further treatment.

10.   **Learn How to Avoid Pain**
    The way you do things may be part of the problem. This science is called Ergonomics, the evaluation of your daily activities. Modifying your behavior and actions may avoid creating some neck problems and headache. Look for more efficient ways to perform your daily routines.

11.   **Do Not Rush**
    Easy does it. Coax your neck to work normally over a few days, even weeks, if needed. Getting used to each new Necksercise takes a little time, some patience and an occasional expletive.

12.   **Function First**
    Make it work. Function comes before comfort. Comfort comes naturally after you restore function. Then keep moving so scars and other tissues will stay loose and not stiffen.

Chapter 5

First Aid—Stop Hurting Now

God helps those who help themselves . . . Proverb

Do It Yourself—Without Work

The following treatments that require little or no effort on your part are called passive therapies. They most often need supplementation with active procedures.

Ice

In the first 24 hours of a problem, ice is great. It works for bruises, muscle tears and acute muscle tightness or soreness from overuse. For a transient problem ice may be all you need to get well.

How Ice Works

Remember how hard it is to smile or talk when you have been out in the cold for a long time. Hawaiians and Southerners, please take my word for it. When the muscles of your face are really cold, they just stop working. To use this reaction, cool the skin and the muscles. The uncomfortable cold feeling peaks just before the skin becomes numb and stops hurting. Cold muscles in your neck cannot work, so they relax. Cold slows pain impulse transmission in your nerves so the area is less uncomfortable. That will let you relax, too.

Ice is safe for just about everyone. Put the ice over a thin cloth or, for some of us with tougher skin, right on the skin itself. Twenty minutes to half an hour of icing should get the area numb enough to be comfortable for several hours. Thicker insulating material takes longer for the ice to penetrate. Rarely, a heavy layer of fat makes the skin too thick; and ice may require more time, or it may never work.

You may repeat icing as often as you need it. Let your skin warm at least once every half hour.

Ice Massage

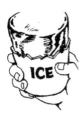

Ice massage relaxes muscles by the pressure of the massage and the cooling effect. Just fill a Styrofoam® cup to the brim with water and freeze it. The ice will expand above the rim of the cup. The cup acts as an insulated handle. As the ice melts, tear the rim back to expose more ice and continue the massage.

If you are a fair-skinned Northern European or an older person, start with five-minute increments. Watch for blistering. Avoid areas susceptible to frostbite such as fingers, nose and toes and by the neck and your ears. Cover sensitive areas to keep them warm.

Use only ice from water or commercial gelatins in plastic cold packs that are labeled "for medical use." *Never* use dry ice for fear of a burn.

Heat

Following overuse or an injury bruises, muscle tears and chronic muscle tightness respond well to heat after the first twenty-four to forty-eight hours. Warmth has been soothing ever since we were cuddled in our mother's arms and, perhaps, earlier. Some things never change. Warmth relaxes not just the psyche but also tired and stressed-out muscles. Muscles become more flexible with increased temperature. Heat also softens the binding tissues of the body including ligaments, tendons and muscle coverings (fascia). This is why you must literally warm up before heavy exercise. Mild heat increases local circulation. Heat helps control infections and helps healing.

Skin and fat are great insulators. If you are "well-insulated," you must maintain heat or ice longer. Moist heat is more effective than dry. Water contains more calories or units of heat than warm air. A warm bath or hot tub transfers more heat in the same amount of time than a sauna. Gentle water massage by active jets also may help distribute heat more quickly. The massage of the jets is a bonus. For the same reasons, a moistened wet-or-dry heating pad is more efficient.

Thin-skinned, fair complexioned people, diabetics and, especially, seniors with delicate skin must consult their physician before using ice or heat.

Keep the heating pad on "low" when used for more than a few minutes.

Is Heat or Ice Better?

Pro Ice

For recent neck injuries or problems ice is safer and more effective than heat. Ice helps control tight muscles or spasm and inflammation like bursitis or tendinitis, but not if they are due to infection.

Pro Heat

For older or arthritic joints, a hot tub, warm bath or shower gives temporary relief from pain and stiffness. Some people prefer the drier heat of a sauna. Perspiration while in a sauna creates a blanket of more efficient moist heat.

Heat, followed by gentle warm-up and light resistance exercises, comforts arthritis patients.

Heat relieves the muscle tightness of nervous tension.

Rest

Rest is a tender trap. Proper rest is essential for good health and normal bodily function. A good night's sleep will relieve tensions produced by hard work. Lack of sleep and unusual or prolonged activity can make you more sensitive to minor discomforts. Injury may follow. Sleep helps healing, but too much rest will not. You need healthy exercise. If you have trouble sleeping, check with your physician. Lack of sleep makes neck pain worse.

After a minor injury or pain in the neck if you can get to work after a night's rest and function well even with some discomfort, do it. You will recover faster when your normal routine is not interrupted.

Rest makes you more aware of your internal feelings like pain. Too much rest creates a downward spiral, increasing pain awareness and decreasing strength and flexibility. Stay active even if it hurts a little and start exercising at any tolerable level. At least go through the motions, then gradually increase resistance and repetitions or time and distance as you feel better. Do your best to avoid deconditioning. That is the medical term for being out of shape. Many physicians observe that a day at bed rest may require a week for recovery.

Relaxation

Once you have relaxed a tight and painful muscle with ice or heat, how do you keep it that way? This is important, especially if your pain is chronic or long-standing. Except for primitive, withdrawal reflexes which are responses to potential injury, you feel and react to pain only in your brain. So, logically, all your pain is in your head. Not funny, just true! Learning how to relax your mind or doing things that let you relax will help. Relaxed muscles will not tense up as quickly or as much.

Tension and stress start in the brain and make pain feel worse. So, the place to reduce chronic pain is your mind, the way you look at pain and the way you feel it. Changing how you react can reduce the impact of pain on your life and function. This is true no matter what the cause.

Learn what helps you to relax. Try music, art, watching clouds, meditation, reading the Bible, the U.S. Budget or whatever it takes. Start relaxing by thinking good thoughts. Then relax your face, eyes and mouth. Continue relaxing your neck and shoulders and arms to your fingertips. Calm your breathing and continue relaxing your trunk and legs.

Dr. Milton Trager was a grand, charismatic doctor, who realized that relaxation helps reduce and even eliminate many musculoskeletal symptoms. He was a clever and honest physician who found a niche in therapy. His forte was to objectify and to teach physical relaxation in an understandable manner.

Eastern philosophers have studied relaxation longer than Westerners. The Easterners developed meditation, Zen, Yoga and other philosophies that promote tranquility. Modern Western behavioral psychologists understand the usefulness of these methods and have copied them. East or West, the idea of "mind over matter" is valid and often useful. Do not downplay this resource as mere mysticism or shamanism. Mental control methods have proven to reduce cancer pain in the terminally ill. If you have chronic neck pain and/or headache, mental relaxation is a good place to begin. Chose the most appropriate guide for you whether it is a guru, minister or a doctor. Professional psychological assistance may be needed.

Chronic pain can cause real changes in the chemical nature of your brain. Do not try to "tough it out." Ignoring chronic pain could change the pain system in your brain for the worse.

Appliances and Aids

Many appliances never have been scientifically proven effective. However, if you try one and like it, then buy it. Most are harmless. Motor massagers tend to reduce pain by confusing the sensory input to the brain. This is also true of the Transcutaneous Electric Nerve Stimulators, called TENS units, which electrically produce the sensation of vibration and partially block pain sensations.

Avoid neck braces, except after surgery or a major neck injury. They have minimal value for most neck problems. They reduce neck activity by getting in the way and promoting pain-focused, avoidant behavior. Remember, function is the key to recovery.

Pillows

Posture is important even when you sleep. Correct spinal alignment at night helps healing and feels better. The pillow must keep your head and neck aligned. Many styles of pillows with different materials are used to hold your 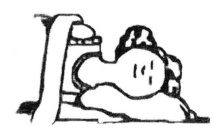 neck in normal alignment. Some are soft. Some are hard. Pillows run the gamut of wooden oriental headrests, the round (Maru) pillow, pillows filled with grains, water, gels and air as well as contoured sponge rubber and the moldable down or memory-foam pillow. They even have temperature-controlled pillows for more demanding customers. Do not forget the speakers under or in the pillow for comforting sounds while sleeping. Comfort, convenience and cost will dictate your choice. Most of these are helpful. Whatever your choice, your head should be slightly elevated and the hollow of the neck fully supported.

Sleeping Postures

No single pillow is right for all bodies. There are three common sleep positions: prone (tummy), supine (back) and side. Each position has different needs for the best head support.

If you do not sleep on your back, at least try to fall asleep that way. As a rule, rolled, horseshoe and contoured pillows work best for supine sleepers. Try placing part of a down or foam pillow under your shoulders to let your head fall slightly, but only slightly, backward. This lets the weight of your head put traction on the neck which may help. If you are a supine sleeper, try a rolled-up towel in the hollow of your neck. This may help you decide on a choice of support.

If you are an inveterate side sleeper, a down or ground foam pillow may be the most practical choice by giving you maximal support in that position.

Chest support using a thin pillow, comforter or body pillow keeps the head from bending too far backward or sideward with prone sleepers.

Better If You Do It Yourself

The other choice besides passive treatment is active therapy when *you* do the work, performing activities that help you get or stay well. When there is a choice, with the exception of properly applied ice or heat, activity should be your first choice for lasting success.

Chapter 6

Okay Baby, Loosen Up!

Failure to prepare is preparing to fail . . . Anonymous

Warm Up Before Stretching

I cannot emphasize enough that your body is more flexible after it is warmed up by activity. Almost any vigorous activity will do. Continue for a minute or two of dancing, running, jumping jacks, pushups or chin ups. Here is one suggestion.

Windmill Warm-Up

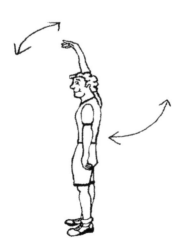

Stand with your arms relaxed at your sides.

Swing your arms back and forth as if walking. Increase the swing until your arms are level with your shoulders at the end of each swing.

Continue for 10-15 seconds until your shoulders feel loose.

To progress, increase the motion by alternately moving each arm through a full circle, so that one arm is up when the other is down, like a windmill. You may need to turn at the waist.

Build up to a full circle slowly, over days or weeks as needed. Avoid this exercise entirely if it is painful

Stretching

Stretching muscles and joints is part of most passive treatments by physical therapists, chiropractic physicians, Rolfers, shiatsu therapists and so on, but you can do it yourself safely, effectively and without any help (or fees) from a professional. Remember, stretching alone is not a substitute for exercise.

- Stretches move your joints through their full range, restoring and keeping flexibility. The tissues around the joints shorten if they are not put through a full range of motion frequently. Even if your pain is from a mild whiplash, the tight painful neck muscles can shrink almost permanently unless you keep stretching them.
- Stretching gives you greater ranges of painless motion by loosening your joints.
- Stretching prevents and reduces muscle pain.
- Stretching prevents injury from sudden and/or extreme movements.
- Stretching not only lengthens the surrounding ligaments, joint capsules and muscles, but it also loosens their blood vessels and nerves.
- Stretching identifies the more painful movements that are caused by tight structures. These are the painful areas that will need more attention when you are actively exercising.

How and When to Stretch

Start your stretches from proper posture with ears in line with your shoulders. If you are sitting, sit up straight and do not slouch.

Stretch at least twice a day to keep loose and flexible. You must stretch more often to restore an injured joint to its full range of motion. The stiffer your neck is, the more often you need to stretch. With age your tissues become less resilient, so you need even more stretching.

Stretch before and after exercise to maintain the ranges of motion you have just developed and to prevent the pain from returning.

Most stretches are held for about fifteen to thirty seconds. Occasionally it may be necessary to stretch a particularly stiff joint repeatedly. Holding a stretch longer causes excessive lengthening called "creep" which should be avoided, as this weakens the over-stretched tissues.

Cautions

- Slow and steady stretching does it every time. Use a gentle, smooth, worm-like movement with only a few pounds of pressure or almost no pressure at all.
- Do not bounce to stretch a muscle or a joint. It is your head on your neck; not a punching bag. Neck tissues can be torn by excessively vigorous stretching. Even a tiny tear will bleed, causing irritation, swelling and more stiffness.
- Do not force the stretch to painful extremes. Most of the action should come from your own neck muscles. For example, tighten the muscles in the front of your neck and bend forward to stretch the muscles in the back of the neck. Apply only light hand pressure on the back of your head for greater stretch.
- Repetition and consistency are the keys to successful stretching.
- Do not do any stretches that cause or increase pain or tingling. Avoid any stretches entirely if it hurts.
- Do not stretch in only one direction. Stretch in the opposite direction for muscle balance.

Try These Stretches

Performing the entire series of following stretches should take only a few minutes.

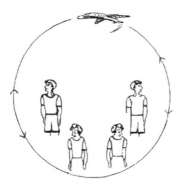

Airplane Stretch

Sit or stand erect with arms at your side or hands in your lap.

Relax and let your head fall forward onto your chest. Then, imagine that you are in a tower watching an airplane slowly taxi and takeoff to the left, lazily climb in the distance, then cross above and behind you, fly far to the right and eventually land in front of you. Reverse direction.

Continue until you feel loose, about 30 seconds.

Nodding Stretch (I definitely said, "Yes"!)

Sit or stand with your arms at your sides or your hands in your lap.

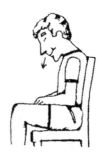

Relax and let your head fall forward onto your chest. Hold for 6-15 seconds.

Repeat once or twice.

Increase the stretch by placing your hands on top of your head and applying gentle pressure

Tick Tock Stretch (Sideways Head Tilt)

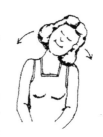

Sit or stand with your arms at your sides or your hands in your lap.

Relax, let your head fall to one side, then try to press your ear toward the same shoulder. Do not lift your shoulder. Hold for 6-15 seconds and repeat in the other direction.

Repeat up to three times.

Ping Pong Stretch (Neck Rotation)

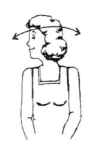

Sit or stand with arms at your sides or hands in your lap.

Slowly turn your chin to look over your shoulder. Hold for 6-15 seconds and repeat in the other direction.

Repeat up to three times.

Chair Pull Stretch

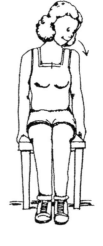

Sit erect with your arms at your sides, grasping the chair and pulling up with both hands.

Slowly turn your head fully to one side while looking down at your chest. Hold for 6-15 seconds and repeat in the other direction.

Repeat up to three times.

Chapter 7

How to Get Better and Not Hurt Yourself

*I wish to preach not the doctrine of ignoble ease, but the
doctrine of strenuous life . . .*
Theodore Roosevelt

Why Should *You* Do The Work?

When there are too many ways to treat a problem, and not just
neck pain, we know that none of them really works well. Just look at
the many head and neck pain treatments: injections, needling, heat
in all forms, ice, pills, shots in the behind and in many other places,
rubbing, pulling and twisting, hypnosis, pressure points, spraying with
coolants and stretching, electric charges, crystals and herbs, liniments,
bracelets and necklaces of different metals and vibrations, burning,
surgery, psychotherapy, several kinds of Yoga and Tae Chi and a host
of proper-named methods like Tragering, Rolfing, Pilates, Alexander
Integrated Balance, Mackenzie, Reiki Touch therapy and that is not
the end.

Exercise is close to a medical cure all. Exercise works, but exercise *is*
work. And, face it, no one can exercise for you. *You* must do the work.
If you stop using your neck muscles they get weaker. Exercise fights this
loss and does a lot more.

Exercise is the safest and best treatment of neck pain and its cousin,
headache. The benefits last longer than any other treatment, and it
works for most people. Exercise permanently reduces neck pain and
often ends the problem entirely.

Exercise is the most effective part of the treatment. Yet, I like the belt-and-suspenders approach and use everything to end your problem, do it faster and keep it from coming back. Ice, some medicines, ergonomics and controlling nervous tension and fatigue supplement exercise like they were meant for each other.

With exercise, you must do it right and keep it up for best results. Necksercises are specific and have an ideal dose and frequency, just like medicines. The right amount and type of exercise is essential to make it work.

Doing It Right

A complete exercise routine includes all of the following to counteract the damage caused by our leisure-loving life style.

- **Maintain flexibility.** Joints need this protection to avoid re-injury.
- **Watch your posture.** Balanced posture reduces the stress on the neck muscles fighting against gravity.
- **Regain Your Strength.** Responsive muscle action protects your neck from the necessary constant and rapidly changing positions.
- **Build Your Endurance.** Increased fitness reduces fatigue and conditions your entire body and brain.

Simple, specific neck exercises (Necksercises) do not need a warning if done properly. However, strengthening exercises need caution, particularly for the ill or elderly. Exercise, if done incorrectly, taken in the wrong dose or performed by the wrong person, will cause injury. Read and understand all the Do's and Do Not's that follow below.

How to Exercise

Stretching for flexibility is most effective when done daily or more often. Stretches are only fifteen to thirty seconds each, so you need only a few minutes for a full routine. The trick is remembering to stretch. Stretching also may restore muscle balance, improve circulation and reduce swelling.

Strengthening exercises are essential for rehabilitation of a neck injury like a whiplash. The goal is to strengthen the neck to normal or slightly higher levels. These exercises improve circulation, strengthen ligaments and improve overall musculoskeletal function even in older people. Strengthening exercises usually are in one to three sets of ten repetitions. Each set is separated by a short rest. You are the judge of what is short. It is usually about a minute.

Resistance exercises are usually done every other day. Daily resistance exercise might be right for you but not for someone else. Each body has its own rhythm or recovery cycle. Respect your body. Feel comfortable for a day before you exercise heavily again. Consistency counts.

Exercise Do's and Do Not's—Review Even If You Know It All

Do's

- Cool ain't cool, Man! You must warm up first. Get your body warmer and more flexible before you tear something.
- Stretch before strengthening. This is the same caveat noted before, but it is even more important with resistance exercises in order to lengthen the tissues around your joints and to give the muscles room to move.
- Stretch your muscles to their proper length. Stretching reduces injuries and painful muscle spasm. Be sure to do it correctly.
- Stretch properly with slow worm-like, painless movements. Do not hurry unless you are looking for an injury as an excuse not to exercise.

Do Not's

- You will make mistakes and get hurt when you are ill, emotionally upset or overly tired. Skip a day of exercise if you are tired or badly out of sorts. Be nice to your body and it will serve you better.

- "Do not rush" deserves repeating. Move smoothly and rhythmically. Enjoy the feeling.
- Bouncing while stretching may cause further injury. Don't be a jerk.
- Feeling good is the beginning of an injury. Resist excesses when you are feeling great.
- Balance proper rest with appropriate exercise.

What to Expect

Exercise is the closest thing to a panacea that we know in healthcare. I know I said that before but it remains true. Here are just a few of the known benefits of good exercise:

- Increasing strength, joint flexibility and resistance to injury.
- Keeping proper body weight, looking good, staying energetic and having endurance.
- Getting more of the brain chemical endorphin that is generated during exercise. This is what makes you feel great and have better endurance. It is the source of the Runner's High.
- Getting better sleep, increasing alertness, improving your appetite, expanding lung capacity, creating a sense of well-being and making life better in general.

There are other suspected, but not yet proven benefits, including:

- Decreasing the occurrence and severity of infections.
- Recovering from infections and injuries may be faster.
- Fighting other diseases may be improved by the hyperthermia of exercise similar to the heat of the sauna.
- Developing better metabolism, improving digestion and even bettering your sex life.

So, do not miss out. You only live once, so why not enjoy life and have more fun!

Working with an Injury

Moderate exercise is fine, but you cannot and should not work through all injuries. This can make an injury worse. If an exercise hurts, you may be doing it wrong. You should re-read the instructions. If your pain still increases with exercise, stop and get professional help.

Beating the Clock with Exercise

Getting in shape has lower and lower limits as we age. You cannot beat Father Time. Sorry, a grandfather can never be as strong and agile as he was when he was twenty-one. With professional guidance, you may push the limits. However, exceeding the limits can bring on serious problems, even death. This warning is probably of little value when talking about the simple Necksercises, or when talking to some knuckleheads about resistance and endurance exercises. The knuckleheads must live and learn.

Chapter 8

Necksercises

Exercise relieves stress. Nothing relieves exercise . . .
Ikkaku, Hosaka and Kawabata in Animal Crossing: Wild
Animal World

ISOMAGIC Exercises for Immediate Relief

Technically, these exercises are called "isometric." I like to call them "ISOMAGIC" because they work like magic. ISOMAGIC exercises restore neck function and give immediate, temporary pain relief. ISOMAGIC Necksercises are advanced first aid for neck pain and headaches.

Basic Instructions for All ISOMAGIC Exercises

- Tighten your muscles, but *do not move.*
- Exercises should be almost painless. If they are painful review these instructions.
- ISOMAGIC exercises are specific and individual for each painful motion.

Starting Position   Identify the painful movement(s). Move your head and neck in the painful direction until it gets a bit more uncomfortable. Then, turn back slightly.

Action	Stop all head or neck movement. Block any motion by pressing your hand firmly against your head, *but never against your jaw.* Press against your hand by tensing your neck muscles and continue to oppose all motion with your hand and arm pressure.
	Hold that position and tension until your neck muscles start to tire, usually more than six and up to twenty seconds.
Hint	If you do not have a watch with a second hand you can count seconds using "one thousand-one, one-thousand-two" or use a single breath for a three-second interval. Three normal breaths would be about ten seconds.
Progression	Remove your hand and turn your neck in the same direction until the muscles start to hurt. Turn back slightly to your next starting position.
Repetitions	Repeat up to five times, advancing your starting position each time.
Variation	Place your elbow on a pad against a wall while pressing your hand against your head.

Adding strengthening or resistance to stretches increases and prolongs their effectiveness compared to simple stretches. You may use hand pressure, gravity, dumb bells, elastic bands or tubing, the weight of your body or machines to accomplish this.

These ISOMAGIC exercises are performed with resistance, *but without movement.* They can be repeated as often as needed. These are my favorites:

Four Corners

Use these exercises when you cannot identify one particularly painful motion or when all movements hurt.

Position 1   Place either hand against your forehead.

Press your head forward against your hand. At the same time, push back with your hand so that no movement occurs.

Hold the pressure for at least 6 seconds.

Position 2   Place your right hand on the right temple.

Press sideways and hold an ISOMAGIC contraction for at least 6 seconds.

Repeat using your left hand on the left temple.

Warning   Press on your temple, not your jaw, to avoid jaw joint pain and damage.

Position 3   Place one or both hands behind your head.

Press backward, but do not allow movement. Hold the pressure at least 6 seconds.

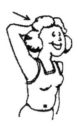

Tighten the muscles but do not move your head from each starting position.

Advanced ISOMAGIC Necksercises

The following ISOMAGIC Necksercises will substitute for "Four Corners" as you get stronger and have less pain.

If the advanced Necksercises are too painful, you are not ready for them. Stay with "Four Corners" for a little longer. Then try advanced ISOMAGIC Necksercises again.

Neck Flexion

This exercise helps when it hurts to bend your neck forward.

Stand facing a wall, two or more feet away. Use a small pad between your forehead and the wall.

Lean your full weight against the wall. Do not use your hands. Keep your neck straight. Hold until your neck muscles tire, 6-20 seconds.

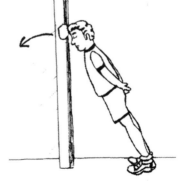

No repetitions.

As your comfort improves, move your feet farther from the wall.

Neck Extension

This exercise helps when it hurts to look up.

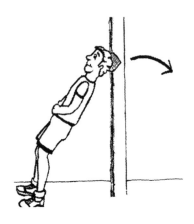

Stand two or more feet from the wall and lean back against a pad or lie face up on suitable padding.

Whether standing or lying, press your head back against the padding. Keep your neck straight. Hold the position for 6-30 seconds

Repeat turning your head partly right then partly left.

As you progress, move farther from the wall. Use a thicker pad if lying down. Turn your head farther right and farther left.

Side Bending

Use this exercise if it hurts to bend your neck sideways.

If it hurts to bend to the left, stand with the wall to your left. Reverse this if it hurts to bend to the right. Step a foot or two away.

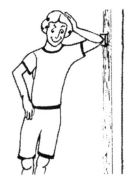

Place your elbow on a pad against the wall. Press against your head while tensing the muscles that tilt your head. Hold until your neck muscles tire, 6-20 seconds.

As you progress, move farther away from the wall and lean your full weight against your hand. Do not use your other hand for support.

Change your starting position by turning your head slightly until the tightest muscle is involved. This increases the effect of this exercise. *Do not move your head during the action.* If the exercise hurts, review the instructions and the illustration to be sure you are doing it correctly.

No repetitions.

Neck Rotation

This exercise helps when it is painful to turn your head.

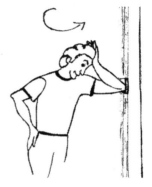

Stand with the wall to your left if turning left hurts. Turn your body a little more away from the wall. Put your left elbow on a pad against the wall and place your palm on your left temple. Turn your head as far as comfortable toward the left. Relax, turning slightly back to the right.

Press your palm against the left temple, blocking all motion with your hand while trying to turn your head toward your hand and the wall. Hold 6-20 seconds until your neck muscles tire.

Repeat up to 5 times, turning your head farther to a new starting position each time as comfort allows.

If it hurts to rotate your neck to the right, repeat the above exercise, substituting right for left. You may need to exercise in both directions.

ISOMAGIC exercises may only give temporary relief. Follow with these exercises.

Isotonic Resistance Exercises

The final goal in stopping head and neck pain is adding exercises with similar resistance through a full range of motion. These are called "isotonic" exercises. Gravity, using the weight of your own body parts, is one form of resistance. These anti-gravity exercises use the weight of your body as resistance and can be done almost anywhere, anytime, without equipment. Adding resistance increases and speeds up return of strength and flexibility. These exercises maintain neck function and comfort and should end your neck and head pain.

Good posture is a key element in correcting and preventing head and neck problems. Isotonic Necksercises strengthen these postural muscles. The combination of ISOMAGIC and isotonic exercises strengthens those muscles even faster, so that good posture becomes automatic.

The goal of these exercises is to perform three sets of ten repetitions, unless otherwise noted. These Necksercises are both therapeutic (if your neck already hurts) and preventive (if you do not want your neck to hurt again).

Shoulder Rolls

Stand or sit with both arms at your sides.

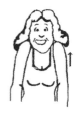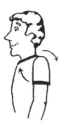

Raise your shoulders forward and up toward your ears. Roll your shoulders back in a circular motion and hold for 6 seconds. Relax and then reverse directions. Do not raise your arms or bend your elbows.

Repeat up to 3 sets of 5 in each direction.

When this exercise is easy, advance to the Turtle.

Turtle (Tillotsen's Shoulder Shrugs)

Sit or stand with your arms at sides.

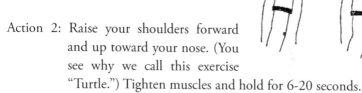

Action 1: Pull your head and chin straight back. Do not tilt your head up or down. This position is very important.

Action 2: Raise your shoulders forward and up toward your nose. (You see why we call this exercise "Turtle.") Tighten muscles and hold for 6-20 seconds.

Note: Action 1 is the most important. If this exercise feels stressful or if you have an acute neck ache or headache, Action 2 may be postponed until you are more comfortable.

Repeat up to 3 sets of 10 each.

To progress, increase the tighten-and-hold position to 30 seconds. Next add weights in each hand. Add one pound at a time, increasing slowly up to 9 pounds in each hand.

You may use a plastic jug with a handle and add liquid gradually. A gallon of liquid weighs about 9 pounds.

The shoulder muscles are essential to movement of the neck. The next few exercises add strength and flexibility to those muscles.

Standing Flys

Sit or stand with your arms loosely at your side.

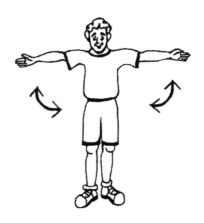

Do not tilt your head. With your palms facing forward, raise your arms sideways level with your shoulders. Hold for 6-30 seconds and then *slowly* let your arms down to your sides.

Repeat up to 3 sets of 10.

To progress, add a weight to each hand, starting with a pound and increasing the weight to 10 pounds as you get stronger.

Pulling a Rope (Shoulder Flexion—Extension)

Sit or stand with your arms at your sides. Hold your head and neck erect, not bent up or down.

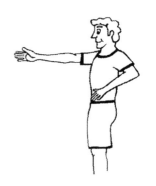

Alternately raise each arm forward to shoulder level. Fully straighten the arm while pulling the other arm down and back in a rowing motion. Hold the end positions for 6 seconds.

Repeat up to 3 sets of 10.

To progress, add a pound to each hand, increasing weight as you strengthen.

Hand position is not important for this exercise.

Look At Your Toes (Supine Neck Flexion)

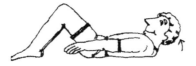

Lie face up on any suitable padding with arms at your side, palms down.

Lift your head off the pad. Hold for 6 seconds and relax.

Repeat up to 3 sets of 10.

To progress, lift your head higher, flexing chin toward your chest.

Prone Neck Extension

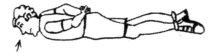

Lie face down on any suitable padding. Place your hands in the small of your back.

Tilt your head back and raise your chin off the pad. Hold for 6-30 seconds and return chin to the pad.

Repeat up to 3 sets of 10 each.

When this exercise is comfortable, proceed to Advanced Neck Extension.

Advanced Neck Extension

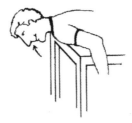

Lie face down on a bench or table with your head over the edge, arms relaxed.

Raise your head level with the table. Hold for 6-30 seconds and relax.

Repeat up to 3 sets of 10 each.

To progress, lift your head while bending your neck farther back.

Side Head Lifts

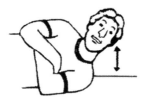

Lie on suitable padding. Turn onto your left side with your arms folded across your chest. Bend your knees for stability.

Raise your head off the pad. Hold for 6-20 seconds and relax. Repeat on your right side.

Repeat up to 3 sets of 10 each.

Chapter 9

Medication and Other Self-Help Treatments

I firmly believe that if the whole materia medica could be sunk to the bottom of the sea, it would be all the better for mankind, and all the worse for the fishes . . . Oliver Wendell Holmes

What Can Medicines Do?

Medications for neck and head pain can make you feel better, but do not cure anything. Medicine is great for minor and passing problems. For most painful problems medicines make it easier to do the necessary exercises.

Remember: All medicines, even natural remedies, can be poisons and have side effects. Some have fewer or more minor side effects than others. Be especially concerned if you tend toward gastrointestinal problems, have allergies and/or have drug sensitivities.

Non-Steroidal Anti-Inflammatory Drugs (NSAIDs)

Many NSAIDs are non-prescription drugs and relieve pain. They are all equally strong in equivalent doses. When taken regularly, NSAIDs also reduce the inflammation that causes the discomfort and muscle spasm from a physical injury, from arthritis or from the chemicals released by a broken spinal disc. Aspirin is the granddaddy of these drugs. Other more common NSAIDs are ibuprofen and Naprosyn®. You can buy many NSAIDs across the counter in slightly smaller than the standard physician-prescribed doses.

All NSAIDs can irritate your stomach, some more than others. To counteract the acid irritation, some medicines are combined with an acid fighter. Medicines like Prilosec® protect the stomach by inhibiting acid production. All NSAIDs have minor occurrences of adverse effects on the cardiovascular system. Check with your physician for appropriateness.

Prescription NSAIDs that may be taken once daily, such as Celebrex® and piroxicam, inhibit a certain enzyme that causes inflammation called COX2 and may have fewer but similar digestive side effects.

Non-Narcotic Analgesics

These drugs control pain and do little else. Acetaminophen (non-aspirin, Tylenol®) is the most popular and safest of the non-narcotic pain killers. If pain relief is all you need, this is the safest drug to use. Rare liver injury and other side effects may occur. It is as effective as aspirin, but without the anti-inflammatory effect. However, it is better tolerated by most adults. Pain relief lasts for several hours, similar to ibuprofen and aspirin. Extended action forms are available over the counter.

Corticosteroids (cortisone)

Corticosteroids are natural hormones that fight inflammation. These are prescription drugs. Corticosteroids often are more effective than NSAIDs, but they can cause more serious side effects, requiring medical supervision. They can lower immunity, delay healing and create sex hormone-like changes. They also cause water retention, muscle weakness, changes in fat distribution, mental disturbances and more problems. Try other medicines first.

Some herbs are claimed to work like corticosteroids. These herbs seem to have about the same good and bad effects as the purified drug itself. Granted, if the effect is weaker (and it usually is) the side effects will be less than the pure drug. Conversely, a smaller dose of the purified drug may have even fewer side effects. An herb contains many different compounds. Unlike the purified pharmaceuticals, these other chemicals present in the herbal medicine may cause unexpected side effects. Finally, there are no clear-cut standards for the strength of herbals, whereas a milligram of cortisone is a milligram, no matter by whom or where it is made.

Narcotics

Narcotics are "controlled substances" like codeine, opium, morphine, Demerol®, dilaudid, Oxycontin® and hydrocodone. These are powerful prescription drugs. They are depressing and addicting. They do not cure anything. Avoid them or use them sparingly as a last resort for temporary pain relief. If you need narcotics for more than a few days, the advice in this book is probably not for you. It is time to work with your doctor.

Muscle Relaxers

A medicine that would relieve tight neck and head muscles would be a boon to modern pharmacopeia. Unfortunately, at the time of this writing, muscle relaxers are a myth perpetuated and promoted to busy health practitioners by some drug companies. This class of habituating medicines is supposed to relax human muscles. However, other than a few experiments on cats, such proof of effective muscle relaxation is only anecdotal. All the muscle relaxants currently prescribed for neck problems act as sedatives or tranquilizers. Nonetheless, these drugs do relax your whole body and your brain and may relax your muscles indirectly.

Personally, I condemn the use of these potentially dangerous, habituating drugs.

Psychotropic Drugs

Physicians may prescribe happy pills (anti-depressants) to help fight the depression of chronic pain. They are generally more effective and more flexible in terms of dosage than over-the-counter St. John's Wort and other naturally-occurring anti-depressants and psychotropics (mind altering drugs).

Some prescription drugs also have a pain-relieving effect by toughening your nerves to pain sensations. Currently these drugs are Neurotin® and Lyrica®. These drugs are being used for more serious and chronic pain conditions. These are rarely needed for most neck pain but may be useful for certain types of headaches.

Cymbalta® is an antidepressant that appears to relieve the strength of pain perception. This use is relatively new.

Finally, psychotropics like amitriptyline help with sleep. Often a good night's sleep is restorative. If you take these drugs you may have to put up with a dry mouth, sleepiness and feeling like somebody else, perhaps with other less common side effects.

Herbs and Nutritional Supplements

Many of today's wonder drugs or their precursors were first found in nature. Quinine, digitalis, aspirin, reserpine and hundreds of others were folk remedies. Drug companies are harvesting newer ones from little-explored forests, molds, strange insects and animals. Yet, only when these drugs are purified, standardized, fully tested and completely documented for side effects, incompatibilities, ideal dosage, dosage in altered health states, shelf life, reliability and after millions of dollars can they be considered ready for the public.

Most often, doctors are reluctant to prescribe herbal medications; because they have not been fully tested for effectiveness and side effects, and the doses are poorly standardized. Using an herbal medication on hundreds of thousands of Chinese over centuries, for instance, does not assure that there has been complete reporting of results and complications. Even though a rhinoceros horn is an interesting phallic symbol, Viagra® is far more effective, cheaper and better for the survival of the rhinoceros.

Doctors and their patients have been burned too often by prescribing drugs that appeared to have been fully tested, only to find that there are devastating side effects. Remember Thalidomide®. To help prevent these tragedies drug companies must spend about $350 million in 2005 dollars to launch a new drug in the United States. And you wondered why Viagra® was so expensive.

Salves and Poultices

The ever-popular poultices, salves, plasters and liniments offer transient relief through two actions. Many are based on a modification of the aspirin molecule which can be absorbed through the skin and, thus, create its usual analgesic effect. These applications also will irritate the skin to bring more blood to that area. Some contain methyl salicylate that smells like wintergreen, others have herbs like menthol, eucalyptol and mint. The increased blood circulation is largely limited to the skin. The irritation or hot feeling confuses the brain. The sensation of warmth in the same area masks the pain, thus making the area less tender. Aspirin by mouth and a warm bath or shower is just as effective and less messy, but it may not be as convenient.

A recent addition to the available topical treatments is the poultice filled with NSAIDs. This method gives a more efficient and direct delivery by plastering the affected area such as an arthritic neck.

Capsicum

Capsicum is the chemical that makes chili peppers taste hot. Unlike the usual liniments and topical applications, capsicum is just a counter-irritant and has no systemic effect. The chemical wears out the pain transmitters in the nerve endings. Penetration of thick skin, heavy muscle and fat and the severity of the pain will limit its use. Capsicum must be applied several times a day. As of this writing this medication appears safer than oral pain relievers, but oral pain medications can be taken at the same time without worrying about incompatibility or overdose of capsicum. The only complication of using capsicum is rare skin blistering, usually due to overuse or improper use with heat or on broken skin or mucous membranes.

Other Self-Help Treatments

The following self-help treatments are purely physical and essentially harmless.

Neck Traction

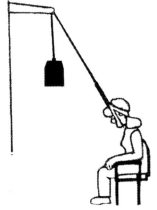

When your neck joints are sore or irritated, your muscles tighten to hold the neck still. Prolonged muscle tightness causes more pain and stiffness. Traction breaks up the cycle of tight muscles causing more pain. Traction is very effective temporarily. Traction lifts the head, relieving the pressure on the sore neck joints and temporarily reducing the pain. Gentle pulling on

Neck Traction

the tense muscles helps them relax. The support of your head and neck lets you relax more.

Traction is simple and is applied many ways. The simplest and most direct is hand traction used by physical therapists and chiropractors and is sometimes combined with manipulation. However, your friend can safely *pull gently* on your neck.

A much safer do-it-your-self method is a relatively inexpensive, over-the-door pulley apparatus. This appliance is available at orthopedic supply stores, but you may need a prescription. The set comes with a head halter and spreader bar to hold your head, some rope and a weight which is often a plastic bag to be filled with varying amounts of water. Traction can be applied while seated, with or without slight neck flexion. Seated position is most convenient, but it requires more weight to equalize the approximately twelve-pound weight of your head. It is more efficient to lie down and relax while traction is applied by hanging the over-the-door pulley on a chair against the bed and pulling straight back horizontally. Fifteen or twenty minutes of traction may give all-day relief and can be repeated as often as you wish.

Avoid any twisting or manipulation by a non-professional. It can be harmful.

Do not put pressure on the chin during traction. The head halter fits under the chin in front and at the base of the skull in back. Slightly change the angle of pull, so the traction bends the neck forward, putting most of the pressure on the base of the skull.

Massage Machines

Mechanical and, especially, hand-held massage devices deliver a quite different effect than manual massage. Deep manual massage aids circulation, tends to relax muscles and causes mental and physical relaxation. Most machines vibrate a light weight that pounds on the sore spot. Others produce non-specific rolling pressure unlike specific manual therapy. The mechanical pounding and rubbing confuses the brain, like rubbing your forehead when you have a headache. The rubbing gives temporary relief as the brain ignores some of the underlying neck and head pain in order to register the rubbing sensation. The pounding and rubbing devices produce mild stretching, but are not as effective as a human hand.

Buddy Massage

If you have someone talented and willing, buddy massage is a great way to reduce neck and head pain. There is no magic to giving a comforting neck massage. Use firm but not painful pressure. Stroke the back of the neck, moving outward and down from the midline of the neck. Continue stroking and/or gently kneading from the head and neck out toward the shoulders and down the upper body. A milking motion also is desirable. Use of a lubricant helps avoid skin irritation.

> Do not use medicated liniments, salves or oils for massaging.

Braces

Some people with neck and head pain complain that their head feels too heavy and that they need a brace to hold it up. Doctors thought that a brace around the neck could help an injured neck heal faster. Neither is true, but these impressions gave birth to the neck collar. Collars can range from bulky sponge rubber to fairly rigid plastic or even metal. Neck braces rest on the collar bones and shoulders and extend to the lower jaw and base of the skull. They are far from comfortable, especially in an August heat wave.

Collars give very little support. They limit neck motion by getting in the way but offer little resistance to an unexpected or forced movement. Collars may be useful for the first twenty-four hours after an acute neck injury or for support after an operation or broken neck. Remove it as soon as your doctor allows. Prolonged wear weakens the unused neck muscles and can injure the jaw joint.

Wearing a collar could become a bad habit. Too often the neck collar is used as a device for $econdary gain, showing the world that the wearer is $uffering in pain, especially following a "whipla$h" injury.

Heat and Ice

Heat and ice are not just for first aid. These are time-honored methods of relaxing tight muscles at any stage of injury. Continue these very useful methods as needed.

Chapter 10

Avoiding Neck and Head Pain

*An ounce of prevention requires pounds of resistance
exercise . . . Dr. Ron*

Prevention is the Best Medicine

Unfortunately, there are severe, untreatable and irreversible injuries
for which we have no solutions. There are diseases of the neck and head
that we cannot cure. Yet, there are many physical problems that can be
foreseen and avoided. The best plan is to do your utmost to prevent
these problems.

The Challenge of Modern Man

Maybe our ancient ancestors should have stayed in the trees.
Nevertheless, here we are standing up on two legs with our heads high
enough to be most effective. We have adapted to being upright, and
it has helped us to survive. But this posture stresses our antigravity
muscles to perform endless fine adjustments for proper balance. The
multiple neck joints require constant monitoring and reaction. Modern
conveniences have made us soft, causing diseases of civilization. One
of the most common of these diseases is deconditioning from lack of
exercise.

Deconditioning

When machines are left idle, they soon stop working and fall apart. The human body is no different in that sense. When muscles and joints are not used, the body rapidly deconditions. Moving parts get rusty. Deconditioned also can be read as out of shape, couch potato or a 150-pound weakling. A couch potato is so accustomed to a seated, supine or prone position that walking and standing become an effort. The weakness continues and affects all activities of daily living. This is deconditioning. Many problems result from this preventable downward spiral of deconditioning.

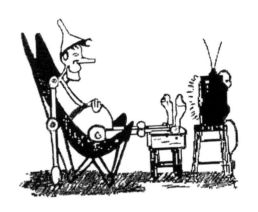

There are many reasons for being well-conditioned besides looking better. The body must be exercised to function efficiently. Neck and other body reflexes are fine-tuned by exercise. Strength reserves are built up to meet emergencies and prevent accidents. As a bonus, exercise sharpens the senses, lowers cholesterol and causes healthful perspiration. Blood supply is increased to the brain for sharper, clearer thinking. Increased body temperature may even help cleanse the body of virus infections. The emotional balance from being conditioned creates a sense of well-being so often absent in a sedentary individual. And, if you have never experienced the sheer joy of a runner's high, a wonderful experience awaits you.

Why Good Posture Is Important

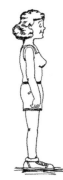

Man needs balance to keep him on two feet. Good posture helps your muscles balance your head. Antigravity muscles struggle to fight the downward pull. (Of course, in the end the muscles loose.) Lower the stress on your neck. When sitting or standing balance your entire body. Do not stoop or slouch. Hold your shoulders back and your head high. Stand and sit tall and stretch for the sky.

Good back posture must be nearly automatic. Think healthy and well-balanced posture. Daily or every other day walk, run, swim, dance or play tennis, basketball, soccer, karate, or do any full-body activity that lasts at least thirty minutes.

Ergonomics

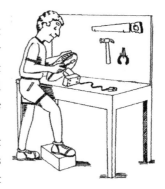

Ergonomics is the science of efficient work, saving energy, preventing injury and lessening the stresses on your body at work or play. Be sure that your work and play environments promote good posture and efficient, balanced movement.

Review the stresses on your body at work. Try to relate your neck symptoms to specific activities and times. A slight adjustment in working surfaces, such as the height or position of a desk, work bench or assembly surface may really help.

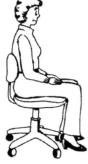

Check your seated posture. Few of us sit militarily erect while working or driving, and even fewer stay that way all day long. Most of the sedentary work force slouches or slumps, aiming the head down and bending the neck forward. If you cannot avoid this position, stand up periodically, roll your head and then roll your shoulders before returning to that punishing, slumped posture. Even if you can sit straight, you need a break.

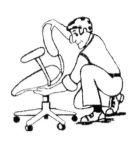

The most sedentary worker can have an ergonomic problem. The ideal chair height for work and study is seventeen inches for the *average* human frame. The *average* desk is twenty-nine to thirty inches high. A secretarial return, the "L" shaped attachment to a desk, may reduce that height by three inches on the *average*. The center of the *average* monitor should be about nine inches higher than the desk surface. But, who and what is average?

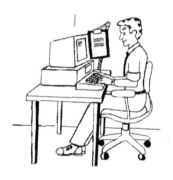

View the monitor from a comfortable position. Adjust your seat height and the tilt or position of the computer screen for the most comfortable head-neck position. Use a chair with adjustable height controls. Raise or lower your seat and/or the monitor instead of craning your neck to see the screen. Consider a copy stand if appropriate.

Adjust your work desk to the lighting or vice versa. Place your computer screen at ninety degrees or a right angle to the brightest, lateral light source. Let the light come from the side. This will reduce glare, eyestrain and tension. If the lights are overhead, move so that they are behind or in front of you, not directly above.

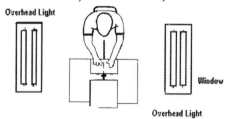

Work, reading and writing surfaces should avoid unusual neck stresses. Place work conveniently in front of you to avoid frequent turning or stressful postures. Good work-surface lighting is essential to prevent that bent-over, squinting posture to see fine print.

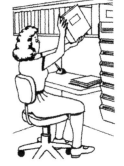

Check special equipment such as meters, controls, monitors, copiers, telephones, treatment machines, files, references, tools and toolboxes, etc., so their surfaces are easy to see and to use.

Frequently-used materials should be within easy reach to minimize twisting or turning.

Check walking surfaces for good traction and proper lighting so that you do not have to watch your feet. Do not be a statue. Move frequently at work or play. Stretch your neck and arms and the rest of your body. Do not stay still for more than twenty minutes at a time. Get up, move and stretch those antigravity muscles. Do a neck roll. Get a drink of water. Look out the window. Move!

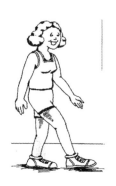

What is your driving posture? Be sure that the car seat is high or low enough to avoid bad neck posture. If the seat cannot be adjusted,

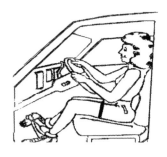

use a pillow. Adjust your headrest. In an accident a properly adjusted headrest could save weeks of neck pain. When seated, keep that curve in your lower back to help keep a normal neck curve. Supporting your feet so that your knees are level with or slightly higher than your hips will help. You might need a footrest or a pedal extension. While you are at it, try a lumbar roll or a pillow in the small of your back.

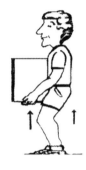
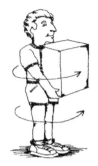
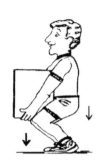

Lift carefully. Balance or counter-balance any weights you carry. Face your work and carry the load close to your body. Use both hands.

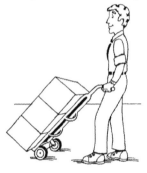

For heavy loads, bend your knees to lift. Keep your feet evenly spaced apart. When turning with a load, pivot your body instead of twisting.

Do not sacrifice your neck or back to save a minute or two. Get help if needed. Use a dolly or hand truck.

Pushing is easier and more efficient than pulling. Push only over level surfaces. Know your limitations and live by them.

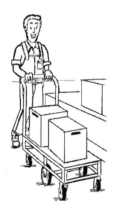

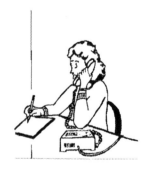

Do not cradle your phone between your head and shoulder for long periods. Use a speaker or a blue-tooth headset.

Unusual positions can cause trouble. For example, avoid lying on your stomach with your head supported by your hands while leaning on bent elbows.

Use a tool belt instead of a tool chest. Shoulder bags can be a problem. Consider a backpack to avoid being off balance. Remember to keep packs light. Heavy backpacks may improve muscle endurance and strength, but they may just as well cause bad posture.

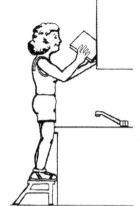

Avoid reaching overhead. Plan ahead and use a stool, a ladder or a lift.

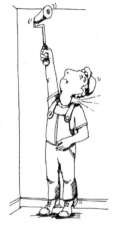

There can be too much of a good thing. For example, some rapidly repeated arm actions may aggravate neck problems. Reduce or avoid repeated gross limb motions required by activities such as lifting, throwing, scraping, painting large surfaces, etc.

Improperly set bifocals or an inappropriate lens may make you tilt your head up or down excessively. This is a frequent cause of a stiff neck. Check your posture while wearing glasses and if you are not in an erect, comfortable position, discuss this with your eye doctor and/or optician (the person who makes the glasses). Consider monofocal contacts or variable lenses for specific tasks.

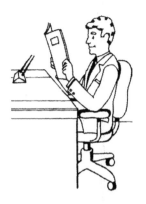

Use armrests or the desk to support your arms while reading. Hold reading material at eye level. Always work with good lighting and a properly adjusted chair. Shift positions every fifteen to twenty minutes to avoid stiffness.

If you read in bed, be sure that your arms are in line with your shoulders and well supported by pillows. Stay erect. Special triangular

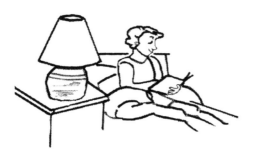

pillows are made for just that purpose. Some even have arm rests. If you are a chronic reader-in-bed, invest in one. Preferably, support both elbows so the reading material will be in your line of sight without bending your neck a lot. Rest your book on a pillow so it is tilted toward you and about fourteen inches from your eyes. The light should be from behind and to one side. When you cannot sit up straight, it is time to sleep.

Body Weight

Some body types pool fat in the abdomen without distributing it equally to other areas. Thus, the abdomen is pulled forward and the pelvis may be tilted downward, making the lower back swayed. This posture causes the hollow in the neck to increase, causing or aggravating neck and head pain.

Wearing your weight around the hips is not as damaging, but in both cases losing weight would be a significant benefit. If you cannot lose weight, build and balance your strength to wear your weight comfortably.

For Women Only

Balanced posture is a further challenge for fashionable women who like to wear high-heeled shoes. The heels elevate but they also tend to thrust the body forward. The trick is to have enough ankle mobility to allow the forefoot to touch the floor without leaning forward. Without a flexible ankle, knees must be bent and balanced by a swayback. When this happens, expect the accompanying backache and neck pain or wear a lower heel.

Some women may have another problem more directly related to neck pain. The weight of heavy breasts can distort posture and create neck problems. Women who are heavy-busted must have adequate support. This can be muscular but a well-engineered undergarment is essential. Rarely, a surgeon may be needed to help if weight loss, strengthening and proper support fail.

Aging and Deconditioning

If you think that deconditioning mimics the aging process, you are right. But a greater part of the change ascribed to aging is not senility but senile thinking. Acting your age is more often the cause of the apparent weakness, lack of energy and enthusiasm associated with aging than the passage of time. Enjoy life by being a participant and not just a spectator. Getting older does not mean you have to sit out every dance. Your body is built to sustain an active lifestyle even as an octogenarian. Do it right and you may be fortunate enough to fall apart all at once far in the future. You can imitate the wonderful one-hoss shay of the Oliver Wendell Holmes' poem which functioned beautifully for many years until it catastrophically and suddenly fell apart all at once.

Chapter 11

Your Choices of Other Passive Therapies

Do not do unto others as you would not have them do unto you . . . Hebrew Proverb

Let Someone Else Do It

Sometimes it hurts too much to do anything that moves your neck. That is when passive treatments can help. Passive therapies are the almost effortless things that you can do or have done *to* you. You just lie back and let it happen. In passive treatment, such as massage, the therapist is the only person getting the lasting benefit of exercise. The patient's benefit is temporary. Other examples of passive treatments are administered by chiropractors, osteopaths, physical therapists and acupuncturists.

Voltaire said, "The art of medicine consists of amusing the patient while nature cures the disease." Even now, over a century later, we doctors are boxed into doing just that. Treating the effect and not the cause leads to this problem. For example, passive treatments will relax tight muscles, the most common reason for neck pain. But you must have repeat treatment until either the problem resolves itself or you tire of the treatment and look for the cause. Here are some of the most effective passive therapies. They are time-honored, safe and temporarily effective.

What Is Passive Therapy?

Until now I have discussed things that you can do to and for yourself to relieve and eliminate your neck pain and headache. However, people often receive only passive treatment for neck pain and headaches from their healthcare providers. This treatment requires that someone do something to you. You become a patient and are dependent on a doctor or therapist to give you relief. Most often passive relief is temporary. Your problems seem to require repeated and prolonged doctor-patient relationships. Some passive treatments may be helpful and smart. But all too often passive treatment becomes a habit—an expensive one. This chronic state of dependency makes you a patient for life!

Many of these therapies are excellent and effective but only when used wisely along with active therapy. Avoid repeated and exclusive use of passive treatments unless you wish to pay for unnecessary lifetime care.

Here are some of the most effective passive therapies. They are time-honored safe and temporarily effective.

Mobilization and Manipulation

Mobilization by physical therapists and massage practitioners moves your joints through a full, normal range of motion. This stretches the muscles and resets their resting length to normal. This is a great idea. The chiropractic, naturopathic and osteopathic physicians accomplish about the same result by manipulating or adjusting as they slightly exceed the normal ranges of motion.

Tight muscles are tight because the muscles are actively contracting and burning sugar fuel. The sore muscles seem to be turned on and will not turn off. All manipulators help reset the tension of your muscles, including the muscles of your neck, by stretching and holding them for a moment or so. By stretching the muscle it learns or resets to a new resting or relaxed length and stops burning up fuel. Burning less fuel more completely reduces the amount of muscle spasm-producing lactic acid, the by-product of the burned fuel.

The cracking and popping sounds of manipulation are satisfying. They may be a signal that the joint has been stretched to its fullest extent and its muscles have been reset to a longer, more relaxed position. These sounds also tell the patient, along with the verbal reinforcement of the manipulator, that something really has been done. In theory, the accompanying gapping of the joint may be beneficial in allowing something to escape that may have been caught, like the lining of the joint. The boney relationships also may be subtly changed or adjusted. Sometimes the patient may feel like a pretzel for a moment or two. However, many patients, including this author, have received temporary benefit as a result.

The osteopathic physician has been taught that his manipulations are more specific than other manipulators. Again, the theory has not been proven but it sounds good. The osteopathic physician has had added training that allows him to legally medicate and operate on his patients.

The manipulative training and technique of naturopathic physicians is similar to chiropractic physicians, but their philosophies differ. These differences often do not change the end result of musculoskeletal-based problems like neck pain and headache. However, it does not make sense to me that one can cure neck pain by treating the opposite end with an enema.

Recent extensive government-sponsored reviews have failed to prove that manipulation by one discipline is any better than the other disciplines. A study published in Spring 1998 by the Rand Corporation think tank, which was funded by chiropractors, concluded that manipulation is a satisfactory treatment for acute or short-term musculoskeletal problems, those lasting several weeks or less, in younger individuals. The corollary is that the treatment should not be extended or repeated ad infinitum, especially in older mature persons.

Stretching: Mechanical and Hands-On Methods

The most direct method of stretching is to pull on the structures to which the muscles are attached. For neck pain these structures are the skull, neck and shoulders. Traction on the neck, by pulling on the head, causes the muscles to stretch, resetting their resting lengths. It also separates the bones and joints of the neck as much as their strong ligaments will allow. Often, this tiny amount of stretch will temporarily relieve pressure against a nerve. It may be all you need to give your body time to heal. This type of stretching can be done manually by someone else or at home with a weight and pulley device. There are many other ways to have your neck muscles stretched including shiatsu, Hawaiian lomi lomi, Rolfing and other deep massage techniques. Twisting the neck also stretches the muscles.

Heat aids muscle relaxation, and many practitioners use moist heat, like warm towels or hot packs, to increase the effectiveness of their massage or manipulation. Practitioners may add electrical stimulation to tire the muscles and, thus, relax them even more.

Relaxation is one key to improving and lowering your perception of pain. Massage feels good and is relaxing. However, as of this writing, there is no evidence that rubbing, pressing, kneading or beating on one's neck and shoulders can help to permanently relieve neck pain or headache. Remember, with the techniques you have learned you can do most of the muscle relaxation yourself with stretches, self-manipulation, heat and/or ice and Necksercises.

Hypnosis

Mind over matter can solve some physical and mental problems, but the technique rarely corrects major health problems. Professional therapists may amplify suggestion or use hypnosis to correct more serious tension-related problems. But hypnosis can be dangerous in the wrong hands. Licensing offers some assurance that the therapist is trained and conscientious. However, in most jurisdictions, hypnotists are not licensed. Caveat emptor!

Psychotherapy

Pain is only perceived by and in the brain. Therefore, the brain should be and is able to control pain. We simply must tap our resources. Often a pain in the neck or a headache is psychological. Persistent tension-related problems may be helped by a psychologist. Most people with chronic pain can benefit from pain behavioral modification therapy. This is especially true if you are more sensitive and tense than average. The behavioral psychologist can train you to handle your pain, so that it does not interfere with your life while you are getting better.

Transcutaneous Electric Nerve Stimulation (TENS)

Pain can be masked by vibration or electrical sensations that mimic vibration with a transcutaneous electric neural stimulator, or TENS for short. An electrical charge passes through the skin to temporarily confuse the nerves that are carrying painful impulses to the brain. The treatment usually is given in an office by a therapist. However, a portable unit can be worn and used intermittently for the same purpose. TENS works for a while. Maybe its effectiveness will last long enough to let your body adjust to whatever problem is discovered or your active therapy can take over.

Trigger Point—Spray and Stretch

Many physicians believe that they can find pain generators called "trigger points." These areas are especially painful when touched or pressed. Some physicians describe feeling a band-like structure in these areas. These trigger points often coincide with acupuncture points.

Osteopathic physicians and others treat these areas by using a cooling spray, sometimes followed by heat, followed by stretching or deep massage. This is a helpful although temporary technique. It is difficult to do by yourself.

Other physicians inject an anesthetic with or without cortisone into multiple trigger points. Many patients tire of this puncturing and opt for other treatments.

Chapter 12

Fire, Needles and Knives

Force is all conquering, but its victories are short-lived . . .
Abraham Lincoln

Invasive therapy is not new. Once treatment penetrates the skin, becoming invasive, the chances of complications and serious damage increase. Ancient physicians practiced brain surgery by trephination to let the evil spirits out of the skull. Some people actually survived this barbaric treatment. Perhaps, our descendants will look upon these modern invasive procedures with similar disdain as we talk about Fire, Needles and Knives in this chapter. There are advantages and disadvantages of each form of treatment. Here are some common treatment methods and some of the risks and benefits of each. Beware!

Palliative Therapies

Some treatments are intended to cure the problem. Other treatments improve the situation but stop short of a cure. These are called palliative therapies and are intended only to make you feel better temporarily.

Some diagnostic tests also are palliative, and therein lies their value in making a diagnosis. If the procedure makes you feel better, the doctor may be on the right track to knowing what is wrong.

Moxabustion

This is a disfiguring, painful, counter-irritant therapy that reminds me of the individual hitting his head against a wall because it feels so good when he stops. It is a mystical Oriental treatment often performed by quasi-religious practitioners with appropriate incantations and by some acupuncturists. An organic moss-like substance, called Mugwort, is set on fire in a small tube-like container on the skin in a location allegedly, either directly and/or indirectly, related to the subject's symptoms. The burning substance causes a small second or third-degree burn about half an inch in diameter which usually heals with a scar. I have seen these disfiguring scars in some of my patients. This would not be my choice for treatment.

Acupuncture

Acupuncture originated in Asia. Oriental medicine is much older than Western medicine's earliest teachers such as Hippocrates, Aesculapius and Paré and, perhaps, even older than the writings of the early Egyptian medical papyri. Although we do not know how it works, acupuncture has proved to be of limited use.

Acupuncturists insert needles into specific areas of the body to influence the natural balance of opposing forces, called Yin and Yang. This is believed to keep the body's life force, or Ci (pronounced chee) flowing properly. Certain sites on the surface of the body, along twelve more or less vertical lines called Meridians, are believed to have relationships to specific organs and regions. Ci when properly channeled or unblocked, the theory goes, can lead to the continuation or restoration of well-being. Electroacupuncture, adding an electric current to the needles, may increase the effectiveness of the treatment. Acupressure activates the classical sites by direct pressure rather than piercing the skin. Westerners, too, often can appreciate the pain relief from acupuncture and its variants.

Acupuncture, electroacupuncture and acupressure each have merit. However, in my experience and that of others, these techniques rarely produce a long-lasting effect, much less a cure. There is a lot of

Oriental theory as to how the acupuncture points generate their desired effects. The reasoning and proof may not satisfy the Western mind. However, objective physiologic changes do result from acupuncture. Acupuncture may relieve pain and nausea as well or better than some medications. Acupuncture with sterile needles seems harmless and is painless, although I was not aware of any benefit when I tried it only a single time. Acupuncture may be a useful adjunct to the treatment of chronic neck pain when combined with exercise. It may work long enough for nature and your Necksercises to correct your problem. Remember, you must restore your function before the effectiveness of the acupuncture wears off.

Trigger Point Injections

In the past several decades an American version of acupuncture therapy has become popular with some medical practitioners. Maybe it is not exactly the same, but to a Westerner it is hard to tell the difference. This technique was championed and popularized by President Kennedy's personal osteopathic physician, Dr. Janet Travell. Western physicians refer to the areas they treat as trigger points. These are very tender and/or painful areas which often coincide with the acupuncture points. Some practitioners believe that the trigger points feel different from the surrounding tissue. Hypodermic needles are used alone or with a local anesthetic and/or cortisone. These trigger points and their mechanism of pain relief are just as elusive of objective scientific proof as acupuncture points, but they have a much shorter history.

Trigger point injections are a real and effective method of pain control for some people and are preferred by certain practitioners, particularly osteopathic physicians and some physiatrists (physical medicine doctor). Numbing the sore area with an anesthetic is often effective in relieving pain for longer than the numbing effect of the anesthetic itself. The effectiveness may be related in some way to the poorly understood acupuncture sites. The injections are rarely, if ever, curative.

Rowlin L. Lichter, M.D.

Diagnostic Tests

Methods have been developed for more accurate diagnosis, both before and during surgery. The MRI helps a lot but is far from infallible. The apparent problem may not be what is bothering the patient. In all cases, corroborating evidence in the physical examination, imaging and electrodiagnostic tests is needed.

Accurately diagnosing the exact source of pain before surgery is critical. Some invasive procedures may be necessary for making the right diagnosis or confirmation of a working diagnosis. Most of these confirming tests will temporarily reduce symptoms.

Epidural Injections

Your doctor may suggest an intra-spinal injection. Usually this is a corticosteroid (cortisone) injection into the spinal canal. If the injection relieves your pain, its major and most important purpose is to let you resume normal activity and exercise before the pain returns. On the other hand, the treatment may last just long enough for your problem to heal itself. This procedure can also confirm that the pain generator is related to the spinal canal. Although complications can be serious, they are very rare.

Joint Injections

Arthritis is a frequent cause of neck pain and headache. Arthritis, by definition, is an irritated joint. Relieving that irritation should relieve pain in that joint. This temporary relief can be obtained by injecting the joint with an anesthetic like Novocain® with or without some cortisone for more prolonged benefit. The injection is a bit tricky but it works. There are no contraindications to taking pain or anti-inflammatory medication at the same time. This type of injection also can be used to find out from where the pain is coming.

Disc Injections

Theoretically, injecting the intervertebral disc can have serious side effects. Although the theory may be wrong, this technique is usually reserved for identifying the exact place to operate. It usually is used in problem cases where there are multiple suspicious areas for the source of pain. The injection is monitored by X-ray. The test is positive if it reproduces the offending pain for a few seconds. A current variation of this test adds an anesthetic and is positive when the injection relieves the pain.

Definitive Therapies

These treatments are intended to be final solutions to cure or correct problems.

Nuking Your Nerves or Radiofrequency Denervation

This technique for combating arthritic neck pain destroys the nerves that carry the pain. Using this method in the low back has received mixed reviews for treating facet joint pain. The equivalent zygoapophysial joints (z-joints) in the neck are at the sides of the cup-shaped structure that fits the upper vertebrae into the lower one. Recent work shows these joints to be important pain generators. If we can find out which of these fourteen neck joints is hurting, killing those nerves might stop the pain. Heating the tissues around the joint with radiofrequency emissions at the end of an inserted needle can destroy these nerves. Because vital structures are so closely packed in the neck, this is too risky to satisfy my comfort level.

Chemonucleolysis

This is an effective but maligned treatment choice. Papaya enzymes or similar chemicals have been developed to dissolve the inside of the disc. Shrinking the disc this way lowers or eradicates the pressure of a bulging or herniated disc on a nerve. This may stop all symptoms. The bad reputation developed from improper use on discs that had broken into the spinal canal. In that case the enzymes injured the very nerves that were to be saved. An additional but avoidable problem is the rare allergic reaction to the enzyme.

Intradiscal Electrothermal Therapy (IDET)

This highly controversial treatment involves heating the center of the disc to destroy its integrity and to let the body absorb it. The procedure may only have a placebo effect as suggested by subsequent investigations. My advice is to wait and try something else.

Surgery

The S word, surgery, may be an option. This ultimate invasive treatment is usually the last resort. It can be a blessing for extreme cases of neck pain but only when properly diagnosed. You must know and understand the benefits and the dangers of the procedure. Asking the doctor how successful he has been with the procedure and how many surgeries he has personally performed is not impolite. There often is a steep learning curve in spinal surgery. The age of the surgeon is not necessarily a good indicator of ability, since some younger surgeons are far better trained than some older ones who have learned on the job. You should know the recovery time and the frequency and severity of possible complications. Considering all alternatives, you may prefer to manage your pain in other ways, since no one has ever died of a stiff neck or headache.

Discectomy is a surgical procedure that theoretically can remove the cause of the neck or head pain by removing the offending disc. If only one disc is abnormal, the chance that it is the cause of the problem is reasonable. Often the diagnosis is not simple. More than one disc may appear sick. Once the disc matures in late teen age, it immediately starts losing elasticity and starts to dry out. By the time one has symptoms of a disc problem, there is often more than one disc that looks unhealthy.

Removing a disc may allow painful motion at that joint. To prevent this, the surgeon may suggest fusing to eliminate the joint. Fusion blocks all motion by replacing the disc with bone taken from elsewhere in the body or from a cadaver. Some surgeons add metal inserts to hold the bone still while healing.

Unfortunately, there are surgical failures. Failed-surgery patients often return for more surgery to remove another disc or to have a fusion. Fortunately, most surgical recoveries take only a few weeks after just a day or less in the hospital.

In the past few years artificial discs have been used to replace the bad ones. Opinions about the benefits of these procedures and styles of mechanical discs are still widely separated. A few of the experimental models appear to be having excellent success. However, there is some concern about financial bias in choosing the right implant. The consensus at this writing is that more work is necessary.

For the desperate, the disillusioned and the unsophisticated there is always an alternative to legitimate therapy. The snake oil salesman will be with us as long as there is a sucker born each minute. We explore the questionable therapies and historical hoaxes in the next chapter.

Chapter 13

Questionable Treatments

The best place for a lie is between two truths . . . The Talmud

Man is quite inventive and his imagination seems limitless. The number of unusual and questionable therapies is far greater than the few I have listed here. Because of the fertility of man's brain, new approaches to symptoms and disease spring up by the dozens each year. Perhaps some will prove to be beneficial like the honey mixture, possibly containing *Penicillium notatum,* which Egyptians placed on wounds according to the 1550 B.C. Ebers papyrus.

Beware: It's a Jungle Out There!

Everyone, Aunt Kate, the barber, Uncle Joe and even the mechanic down the street, has an answer to your neck problem from Grandma's kitchen, or something pseudoscientific to maybe even a little professional.

Almost everyone means well. However, some health merchants sell fancy buzz words like organic, vibrations, harmony, symbiosis, biotic and my favorite, holistic medicine. They pervert the word holistic to mean using herbs, diet, divine intervention, mysticism or Ci to cure disease. Holistic just means treating the whole person, mentally, spiritually and physically. Good health practitioners do this all the time, but maybe not all of us are good ones.

You often can pick the hucksters out of the legitimate practitioners by some of the usual things they say and do. They usually avoid standard medicine practices and downplay the standard methods of care. They may indicate that the American Medical Association is against them unfairly. (The AMA may never have even heard of them.) They describe miracle cures. They usually demand concurrent or prior payment. Their wallpaper (diplomas) is from obscure institutions. They rely heavily on personal stories of success, such as promotions by a health practitioner and his followers who made diagnoses of diseases not found by licensed physicians and cured patients after expensive treatments. Finally, hucksters often will list obvious truths and include a false theorem or view that seems to support their deceitful claims. Be vigilant against deception.

Manipulation helps, but too often it can be abused. Temporary relief requires frequent return visits, sometimes extended for months or years, creating physician dependency. In other words, you needlessly become a patient for life. When you need manipulation it is smart to sharply limit your treatments or, better, do it yourself when and where you need it. It is also a lot less expensive if you do it.

The following is an objective evaluation of each of the listed therapies. You decide whether a Pasteur or a Barnum is running the show.

The Placebo Effect

Placebos are the most pervasive of all therapies. For the most part they are harmless and are estimated to be effective in a quarter of the cases. If one is convinced that a treatment works, it has a better chance of being effective. This is so strongly true that medications such as salt water, sugar water or colored lights and amulets can improve and even cure real disease and injury. Approximately two-thirds of all physicians and health practitioners use this effect.

Many diseases are caused by the patient's own mental concepts. When this illness behavior is changed, either by education, conditioning, hypnosis or trickery, the patient is cured.

Unfortunately, this wonderful tool is easily manipulated to the advantage of the charlatan. The negative side of the equation is just as simple to emphasize. An unscrupulous health practitioner can convince a patient of the need for prolonged care and dependency by verbal reinforcement, impressive but useless machinery or soothing physical treatments of questionable or transient value.

Suggestion

Suggestion is a close companion of the placebo effect and is the basis of hypnosis. All of us are suggestible to some degree. With proper training the effect of suggestion can become almost a command. When this power of the mind is used for health, to end a bad habit for example, it is a great therapeutic tool. Reiki Touch Therapy is probably a good example of the use of suggestion. When it is used to convince a patient that he or she must have a particular therapy to remain healthy, it is a tragedy. Unfortunately, this misuse of a powerful tool is a very familiar scenario in modern health care.

Get a second opinion if your neck problem requires seemingly endless periodic treatment for flare-ups, maintenance therapy or multiple recurrences or aggravations. You could be a victim of negative suggestion, habituation or enforced physician dependency.

Snake Oil Remedies

If it sounds too good to be true, it probably is not. Beware of cures that allegedly have been suppressed by the American Medical Association. Doctors and their families have health problems just like everyone else. If something could cure them or their families, they would be near the head of the line demanding it. As medical doctors we have taken an oath not to withhold reasonably effective therapy, but we do condemn charlatans. The logic of many unproven cures is usually anecdotal or unscientific testimony without a proven scientific basis. Documentation usually is poor and questionable. Many of these procedures are useless, and some could be harmful.

Remedies with Testimonials

Testimonials often are powerful persuaders. The apparent success of a treatment strengthens the placebo effect that usually helps up to twenty-five per cent of patients. This success rate can make a good living for someone. Saying it another way, one out of every four people is pleased by sugar pills. The three others who fell for the pitch probably are too ashamed to demand their money back.

Foreign Medicine

Do not seek care across a border where licensure and treatment are not well controlled or policed. The practice of medicine in many foreign university medical centers is excellent. However, some foreign practitioners have been known to use dramatic but dangerous drugs such as phenylbutazone and high doses of cortisone that produce short-lived and dramatic improvement of arthritis with possible disastrous side effects. These doctors may use drugs banned in the United States because they have caused death or serious side effects. Medications may not be approved by the Food and Drug Administration or may be prescribed in unsafe doses. There is no assurance of quality in any medical degree, but a license to practice in the United States offers a greater degree of insurance than most granted elsewhere.

Foot Massage or Reflexology

Foot pressure-point massage has been touted to cure all sorts of illnesses with specific pressures in specific areas affecting all sorts of remote functions. The procedure has been given stature with the name Reflexology. Localized foot pressure, like stepping on a pebble or wearing tight shoes, has no provable remote consequences. On the other hand, if the placebo effect of foot massage makes you feel better and you can afford this type of treatment, go for it. Oops, I just stepped on my kidney!

Copper, Magnetic or Tuned Bracelets, Pendants or Amulets

These have the same effects as any other magic charm. They are as effective as one's belief. The amount of copper absorbed through your skin is insignificant. Magnetism and frequencies are useless. Even if a significant amount of copper were absorbed through the skin, there is no evidence that copper in any form is therapeutic for nerve or joint problems. In fact, copper compounds are inherently poisonous. However, if the problem is related to tension or a mental attitude, any form of therapy can be effective if the patient believes that it will work.

Shark Cartilage, Glucosamine, Chondroitin, Methylsulfonyl Methane (MSM)

These dietary supplements are supposed to help restore the cartilage of arthritic joints. Some neck and head pains are related to arthritis. The arthritic joint has lost cartilage. But, eating cartilage or its components to restore the joint cartilage is as useful as drinking blood for anemia or eating brains to get smarter. The stomach and intestines are indiscriminate in digesting proteins, complex sugars and fat whether they are derived from blood, brains or fish—even sharks. So far, eating shark, cow or pig cartilage appears to be useless despite the 1996 published claims in *The Arthritis Cure . . .* by Theodosakis and Buff which was revised and updated in 2011. In most cases, the few extra calories of food value are all that would be gained. The extra money you pay for these supplements is your loss. Since arthritic symptoms vary from time to time, some reinforcement of the placebo effect is not unusual.

Despite this discussion, there may be some objective evidence in a controlled study that glucosamine, a breakdown product of cartilage or some part of it, may relieve the symptoms of osteoarthritis. The chondroitin found with glucosamine in cartilage may have no therapeutic benefit. However, many prescribers have no qualms about recommending the chondroitin-glucosamine complex.

Remember, doctors have painful osteoarthritic conditions, too. Ask your doctor what he or she uses.

Prolotherapy

Physical or chemical insults can produce stiff scar tissues. A few practitioners believe in this old, unproved theory which was revived in the 1940's by George S. Hackett, M.D. When a joint moves excessively or painfully in its normal ranges of motion, reducing this motion will reduce pain. Nowadays the practitioner attempts to limit the motion by creating a tough scar with sclerosing (scarring) solutions.

Prolotherapy superficially seems like a reasonable theory. However, as with many theories, it dies with the execution. The problems are (1) it is difficult to produce a significant limiting scar around a joint without further injuring the joint, (2) it is impossible to predict exactly where and how much scar will be produced and (3) what will the scar do? This is essentially a crap shoot with the bet being your health and comfort. My advice is to avoid this procedure that has not gained favor in over fifty years. However, this method has been used successfully for one condition. An ancient Roman cure for dislocation of the shoulder was to use a red-hot poker to sear the deep tissues in the front of the shoulder, creating a scar that kept the shoulder in the joint. Fortunately, the procedure is rarely suggested for the neck.

Craniosacral Therapy

This is an unusual variant of osteopathy that makes even the heads of most osteopathic physicians shake. The skull is composed of several bones that are welded together by saw-tooth-like joints stuck together with tough nylon-strong collagen fibers. This unusual theory holds that a diseased state is caused by skull bones moving almost imperceptibly to produce improper pressures on the brain. The procedure requires several practitioners to simultaneously apply carefully directed hand pressures on the patient's skull. While one or two practitioners press a pair of skull bones toward each other, a third practitioner presses or lifts another offending cranial plate to reposition it into its normal relationship. Most physicians believe that it is impossible to diagnose the minute displacements that the proponents claim they are correcting. Having three doctors with six hands pressing on your skull in unison with appropriate accompanying remarks must exert a strong suggestive influence on your perception of your complaints. Personally, I would avoid this treatment at all costs. With three doctors working on you at the same time, those costs would probably be well worth avoiding.

Magnets

Attractive theory or not, curing disease with even the strongest magnets available is nothing short of ridiculous. Nonetheless, the gullible public has made the sale of these useless gadgets quite lucrative. The MRI used many times a day in thousands of clinics throughout the world produces far more magnetism without a therapeutic or significant physiologic effect than these toys. The real part of the magnetic cure is the conviction of the snake oil huckster. P.T. Barnum is famous for popularizing a gambler's statement that "There's a sucker born every minute." It is a lucrative business.

Rolfing

Rolfers theorize that their deep massage therapy, which is alleged to be painless, is able to move the nylon-strong connective tissues of the body to a healthier, balanced position. As a surgeon, I have attempted to manipulate these connective tissues to see deeper structures. The strength of these tissues makes it difficult to believe the Rolfers' theories. You may be more comfortable after this deep massage, and you may be wise to follow some of the health advice which accompanies the treatment.

Radon Mines

Radon may be one of mankind's oldest therapies, documented as long ago as 6,000 years. For more than eight centuries Japanese have been visiting radon therapy clinics and underground galleries in the hopes of curing arthritis and other diseases. Now we clearly understand the dangers of radiation. In fact, today there is a thriving business in radon detectors so we can avoid the gas. However, current treatment at one facility in Montana indicates that the radiation exposure for thirty-two hours over ten days is insignificant.

I wonder how many of today's treatments will be considered ridiculous in the future?

Chapter 14

Finding Professional Help

A doctor who treats himself has a fool for a physician and an idiot for a patient . . . Anonymous

Using the program outlined in this book your headache or neck pain should improve day-by-day. If your symptoms do not improve progressively over a few weeks or if the cautions outlined earlier occur, it is time to seek professional help.

What are your choices? How do you find someone who is right for you?

Self-Diagnosis and Self-Medication

Self-diagnosis and self-medication are dangerous. Not the least of these dangers is making a bad diagnosis and delaying treatment of a serious disorder that may have been more easily corrected earlier.

Choosing a Medical Doctor

In today's alphabet soup of health care, your first step will be to see your family doctor or his equivalent; i.e., The Gatekeeper or Primary Caregiver. When the practitioner learns that your pain is not improving, he or she should refer you to a specialist. If you have followed the advice of this book, you should not need a referral to physical therapy. The rare exceptions are those people who have tried to exercise but failed. They may need the guidance and encouragement of a professional in the structured environment of a physical therapy or rehabilitation facility.

The specialist should be in one of six fields: physical medicine, orthopedics, neurology, rheumatology, neurosurgery or psychiatry/psychology.

Physical Medicine specialists are called Physiatrists and may give medicines and injections along with prescribing exercise when indicated. Some patients are delighted to know that these practitioners never operate. Orthopedic Medicine specialists are similarly trained.

Orthopedic Surgeons treat bone and joint diseases and injuries that are largely due to surgically-correctable problems. They often work hand-in-hand with the non-operating specialists.

Neurosurgeons diagnose and operate on problems of the brain, nerves and spinal cord. They are appropriate for neck injuries with arm pain or severe, relentless headaches.

Neurologists diagnose the problems treated by a neurosurgeon or an orthopedic surgeon. They, too, do not operate. You may wish to see a neurologist first.

Rheumatologists treat diseases of the muscles and joints and do not operate. They may diagnose a surgical problem and refer you to a surgeon or they may prefer a physiatrist for follow up.

Psychiatrists are medical doctors who help you mentally conquer pain. They may add medication and give injections to help.

Psychologists are not medical doctors but are adept in leading you through steps to conquer your pain through mental exercises.

Once you have selected the right specialty, ask about the doctor's credentials, experience and outcome history. You should know how much experience the doctor has had with your kind of problem and just how successful his patients have been with the chosen therapy. You have a right and a need to know the quality and extent of the doctor's training and experience. Choose your caregiver carefully.

In the modern setting of HMOs, PPOs and other alphabetic administrations, it gets harder and harder to find a friendly, concerned treating physician who is willing to listen. A well-educated assistant to the doctor may be your only choice. Do *not* leave the doctor's office with unanswered questions. You have a right and a duty to know what is happening to you and what your future or prognosis is. A good practitioner can give you a suitable and understandable time table. You must be part of the therapeutic team and be fully informed.

Check the doctor's wallpaper. The diplomas that hang on the wall tell you where and how well the physician has been trained. Do not hesitate to ask. You are paying for his or her services, and you have a right to know how good those services promise to be. Does the doctor teach at the local medical school? The challenge of students most often sharpens one's skills. To what hospital staffs does he belong? Hospitals, especially university-affiliated teaching hospitals, are very strict about maintaining high professional standards. Does the doctor maintain his educational expertise? Board-certification diplomas may be displayed in the office. Does the doctor belong to some of the exclusive medical sub-specialty societies that require further education and testing?

Complementary and Alternative Medical (CAM) Practitioners

Selecting an alternative health practitioner is a reasonable option. Such drug-free treatment can and should be continued as long as improvement continues. Be cautious if your problem repeatedly recurs.

Many chiropractors have been taught and assume that the nervous system has been blocked by malpositions of the spinal column (subluxations) and manipulate (adjust) your body to restore healthy relationships. When choosing a chiropractor you may choose a straight or a mixer. The straight chiropractor does not believe in the need for or effectiveness of medicines or surgery and understands that blocked nervous energy is the sole cause of all disease. Mixers are, to varying degrees, amenable to the concept of bacterial and viral sources of infection and the effectiveness of antibiotics and other pharmaceuticals in controlling or curing disease. A distinct benefit of Chiropractic Medicine is that no chiropractor has ever produced a drug addict or a failed surgical result, and they have a fair batting average in controlling neck pain and some headaches.

Homeopathic physicians are recent revivalists of Socratic medicine which cured diseases with infinitesimally small doses of medicines that produce the disease symptoms in their higher doses. The homeopathic physician has been taught that almost pure water with almost no medication is the strongest cure when matched to the disease.

The Naturopathic Physicians understand that nature will cure the disease with a little non-chemical help such as herbs, cleansing enemas and manipulation.

Osteopathic physicians were originally taught that the major causes of sickness were related to boney malpositions, but now they primarily follow allopathic (medical doctor) ideas. Most of them use manipulation only as a small part of their treatment.

Practitioners of Eastern Medicine and Herbalists fill out this list of choices but do not complete it. There are many more choices including touchers, rubbers, mentalists and faith healers. See Chapter 13.

What to Expect from Your Doctor

You and your doctor will try to determine just what is wrong. Allopathic physicians (M.D.s) will try using scientific concepts and anatomic terms. Most of them will order x-rays of your neck, looking for old or new injuries, arthritis, congenital abnormalities, new growths or infection. Except for advanced arthritis or fractures, these x-rays will rarely find your problem. Most doctors have their favorite first tests. A rheumatologist may order blood tests, looking for arthritis of one kind or another. The neurologist or physiatrist may begin with needle electrode studies, looking for impaired nerve function.

Besides taking a history, examining your neck should include:

- Your neck motion limitations and pain
- Muscle tension, strength and tenderness
- Function of the nerves of movement and sensation and special senses
- Your state of physical conditioning
- Some tests for circulatory problems
- Your jaw for joint problems

- Headaches may require further tests such as brain imaging or EEG (Electroencephalography).

Above all, the doctor must get to know you and what makes you tick, both physically and emotionally.

If your symptoms persist, most doctors will eventually order Magnetic Resonance Imaging, an MRI. A person is placed in a super magnet and is rapidly magnetized and demagnetized. It is hard to believe but true. The changing magnetism causes the water in the body to give off radio waves that are mapped like radar, but in three dimensions. The map shows the differences in water densities inside one's body. Since most tissues have different amounts of water, we can see each structure separately as a different shade of grey. The test is harmless but is noisy and confining. It may take about an hour of lying still. All patients are screened by x-ray for metal in the eyes. Because any magnetic material in your body may interfere with the test and may wander dangerously if the magnet moves it, an MRI is not an option for patients with metal fragments and metal implants like pacemakers. The alternative, Computerized Tomography (CT) Scan, is almost as diagnostic.

After your doctor reviews the tests, he should explain your diagnosis. Learn what can be done for your problem. How successful is each method of treatment? What happens if you do nothing? Doing nothing is always an option. Sometimes it's the smartest one.

If the doctor prescribes medication such as NSAIDs, learn the possible side effects and incompatibilities. Ask about alternative medication. Avoid long-term use of narcotics, even mild ones. All narcotics are habit-forming and some are addicting. You do not need another problem.

Expect a similar succession of events when you see physicians of alternative or complementary medicine. But each health care practitioner will emphasize different aspects of the diagnostic and therapeutic plans. A chiropractor may delve into intricacies of your x-ray. The homeopathic physician may investigate your mood and emphasize the exact nature of your symptoms. Practitioners of Eastern Medicine may look at your eyes and skin while carefully feeling you pulse. Each practitioner adds his or her own tests and procedures and leaves out some that other practitioners would order or perform. Nonetheless, they all are treating the same organism, you, which requires the same attention to your needs while avoiding injury. Delay in treating a serious disease could be dangerous no matter which discipline of health care you chose. Expect and demand as much or more in terms of diagnosis, treatment and improvement from an alternative health care practitioner as you would from an allopathic physician.

So-Called Flare-ups

Recurrence of symptoms is often disguised as a "flare-up." Remember, a dead fire will not flare up. This is simply a cover-up for inability of the practitioner to cure or fully control your problem. You may choose to live with incomplete control. You also may seek a more appropriate and effective treatment.

Epilogue

I truly hope that this book has been of service to you. In my broad view of many decades, medicine has changed from the meditating family doctor illustrated by Norman Rockwell to the highly specialized scientist supported by almost unbelievable technology.

Even more difficult for me to understand is the popularity of ancient treatment methods and theories with a significant number of informed people despite the growth in accuracy and effectiveness of the science and practice of modern allopathic medicine. There are hundreds of thousands of people in the Americas and a huge number more in the Indian subcontinent who follow and practice Ayurvedic medicine. There are uncounted numbers in the Americas who follow Amerindian Shamanism. I have had no direct experience with either method. Each culture and many subcultures throughout the world have continued to support folk medicine in significant numbers. For *Stop Your Neck Pain and Headache Now* to cover each of these systems would have required an encyclopedic expansion.

The past persists, and although the present dominates what does the future hold? It is inevitable that tomorrow will be different. I have seen treatments which were fully accepted and universally followed by allopathic physicians suddenly become anathema following new scientific evidence. The principles I espouse as basic are based on today's science, but they may fade into obscurity or even be condemned tomorrow. For example, in orthopedic surgery in the 1950s we would remove a torn anterior cruciate ligament of the knee because it interfered with movement. Today we feel this is abhorrent and do everything possible to reconstruct this essential ligament. This is only one of many earlier misdirected treatments that we fully accepted in orthopedics only to be considered injurious today. So, in this ever-changing area of science nothing is written in stone.

The methods and advice in *Stop Your Neck Pain and Headache Now* have been repeatedly tested by me and others for decades and appear to be reasonable and effective. However, as pointed out in my ligament illustration above, things change. Therefore, note the date of publication of this book. Know that the process of writing and publication adds to the age of printed material and that the material presented was based on then current knowledge. I have done everything reasonable to make these writings current, but facts will change. Be aware that the truth, unfortunately but honestly, will change from time to time.

As a corollary, never follow your physician's advice blindly. There are many well-traveled paths in medicine, even in modern medicine; and they may not all lead to successful results. Understand what is being asked of you or proposed to be done. Question your practitioners and demand concise answers as well as alternatives. Even a truthful "I don't know" might be acceptable.

One person cannot be the ultimate authority on anything. If what is required of you or what you are advised to do does not make sense, ask another authority. Then you must be the judge. It's your body. Take your stewardship seriously.

Thank you for your attention. I hope you have enjoyed reading this book as much as I did writing it. Let me know how you like it at dr_ron@nvbell.net. With your suggestions and the progress of medicine I hope to write a second edition as we learn more about how to *Stop Your Neck Pain and Headache Now.*

Please use this book in good health. If this book has helped you, consider passing it on and sharing it with a fellow sufferer.

About the Author

Rowlin L. Lichter, M.D., is a board-certified orthopedic surgeon trained at Northwestern University with more than sixty years of clinical experience. A pioneer in sports medicine, Dr. Lichter established the prestigious CHART Rehabilitation Centers of Hawaii in 1979. He now donates his services to the underserved in Reno, Nevada. The parents of five children, he and Barbara, his wife of almost fifty years, share a love of food, wine, travel, and writing.

Index

Rowlin L. Lichter, M.D.